Nuclear Medicine Therapy

Luca Giovanella

Editor

Nuclear Medicine Therapy

Side Effects and Complications

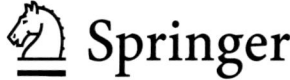 Springer

Editor
Luca Giovanella
Nuclear Medicine and PET/CT Centre
Oncology Institute of Southern Switzerland
Bellinzona
Switzerland

ISBN 978-3-030-17493-4   ISBN 978-3-030-17494-1   (eBook)
https://doi.org/10.1007/978-3-030-17494-1

This Springer imprint is published by the registered company Springer Nature Switzerland AG
The registered company address is: Gewerbestrasse 11, 6330 Cham, Switzerland

To our patients and their families for giving meaning to our work.

Preface

In the last two decades, the demand for a personalized therapeutic approach has been constantly increasing, mainly due to the need to develop ever more effective therapeutic regimens, to improve outcome, and to avoid unnecessary treatments. Theranostics is an invaluable tool in personalized medicine; it is a treatment strategy in which the same (or very similar) agents are used for both diagnostic and therapeutic purposes. Particularly, theranostics is based on the integration of a diagnostic test and a specific treatment, and it relies on the idea of selecting patients through a diagnostic study that could detect whether a patient will benefit from a certain therapy or not.

Nuclear medicine is ideally placed to play a central role in this field by allowing visualization of molecular targets and thus enabling so-called in vivo immunohistochemistry, by which noninvasive biomarkers can be provided to select targeted drugs labeled with therapeutic radionuclides. The theranostic procedures are based on radiolabeling compounds of interest and performing tailored low-dose molecular imaging to provide the necessary pretherapy information on biodistribution, critical organ or tissue, dosimetry, and the maximum tolerated dose. If the imaging results then warrant it, it would be safe and appropriate to follow up designing higher-dose targeted molecular therapy with the greatest effectiveness and safety.

Holding a wide and in-depth knowledge of the advantages and disadvantages that ensue from the application of theranostics is an essential requirement to properly exploit this tool in clinical management. Conscious of its limits, theranostics can be successfully applied as a powerful strategy in cancer treatment, and nuclear medicine owns the tools to play a central role in this field. Our scope is to provide essential but exhaustive information on nuclear medicine theranostics with emphasis on clinical management of side effects and potential complications.

Bellinzona, Switzerland   Luca Giovanella

Contents

Nuclear Medicine Theranostics: Between Atoms and Patients

Alice Lorenzoni, Antonella Capozza, Ettore Seregni, and Luca Giovanella

In the last two decades, the demand for a personalized therapeutic approach has been constantly increasing, mainly due to the need to develop ever more effective therapeutic regimens, to improve outcome, and to avoid unnecessary treatments. Theranostics is an invaluable tool in personalized medicine; it is a treatment strategy in which the same (or very similar) agents are used for both diagnostic and therapeutic purposes. Particularly, theranostics is based on the integration of a diagnostic test and a specific treatment and it relies on the idea of selecting patients through a diagnostic study that could detect whether a patient will benefit from a certain therapy or not [1, 2].

Allowing the stratification of patients into those responding and likely to respond to the therapy and those better treated in another manner, useless and time-wasting therapy can be avoided. A step forward, from personalized therapeutic pathways, is represented by the individualization of treatment. Although a fixed approach to therapy may be more practical, an individual-ized approach is more likely to ensure that each patient receives an effective drug and drug dose that has acceptable and definable tissue effects, keeping the highest safety margin [3].

A theranostic diagnostic agent should enable the disease localization and state, as a surrogate for a potential therapeutic agent with similar chemical properties; should allow the examination of its biodistribution as predictive of off-target (adverse) effects of the potential therapeutic agent; should be useful in determining the optimal therapeutic dosage or activity to be administered, based on the predictive tumoricidal doses measured in the tumor site; and should be useful in monitoring treatment response [4, 5]. This concept is not specific to radiopharmaceuticals but is easily applicable in nuclear medicine. Personalized genomics, proteomics, and molecular imaging are among technologies currently used for theranosis.

Nuclear medicine is ideally placed to play a central role in this field by allowing visualization of molecular targets and thus enabling so-called in vivo immunohistochemistry, by which noninvasive biomarkers can be provided to select targeted drugs labeled with therapeutic radionuclides [5]. The theranostic procedures are based on radiolabeling compounds of interest and performing tailored low-dose molecular imaging (single-photon emission computed tomography/computed tomography SPECT/CT or positron emission tomography/computed tomography PET/CT) to provide the necessary pretherapy information on

A. Lorenzoni · A. Capozza · E. Seregni
Nuclear Medicine Unit, Fondazione IRCCS Istituto Nazionale dei Tumori, Milan, Italy
e-mail: alice.lorenzoni@istitutotumori.mi.it;
antonella.capozza@istitutotumori.mi.it;
ettore.seregni@istitutotumori.mi.it

L. Giovanella (✉)
Clinic for Nuclear Medicine and Molecular Imaging, Oncology Institute of Southern Switzerland, Bellinzona, Switzerland
e-mail: luca.giovanella@eoc.ch

© Springer Nature Switzerland AG 2019
L. Giovanella (ed.), *Nuclear Medicine Therapy*, https://doi.org/10.1007/978-3-030-17494-1_1

biodistribution, critical organ or tissue, dosimetry, and the maximum tolerated dose. If the imaging results then warrant it, it would be safe and appropriate to follow up designing higher-dose targeted molecular therapy with the greatest effectiveness and safety [4].

The theranostic approach finds its main application in the oncology field. Cancer is an extremely heterogeneous disease, as it varies from patient to patient and it might include, in the same individual, a diverse collection of malignant cells harboring distinct molecular signatures with differential levels of sensitivity to treatment [1]. This heterogeneity might result in a nonuniform distribution of distinct tumor-cell subpopulations across and within disease sites or temporal variations in the molecular makeup of cancer cells. Heterogeneity is the source of resistance to treatment; all accessible therapies are effective for only limited patient subpopulations and at discriminatory stages of disease development [6]. Therefore, an accurate characterization of tumor is essential for treatment planning and targeting approaches are gaining increasing interest.

Designing a specific targeting/killing combination is a tailoring process. Significant and rapid advances in molecular biology continue to lead to a better understanding of cancer, and many biological vehicles, such as monoclonal antibodies, specific proteins, and peptides, have been identified. A variety of molecules has been designed to serve as systemic carriers, able to selectively deliver imaging photons to diagnose disease, or therapeutic electrons to deliver cytotoxic radiation, in a highly localized manner. These developments have led to a renewed interest in the possibility of treating disseminated malignancies with the systemic administration of radionuclides [4]. In this scenario, theranostics finds a soil to grow.

Although the term has been coined recently and theranostics is proposed as an innovative approach, the concepts underlying theranosis are not new at all in the field of nuclear medicine and have been applied in patient care for almost a century. Detecting and targeting a pathological process, using the same or at least very similar molecules (tracer), either labeled with different isotopes or nuclides or given in different amount, in order to identify, diagnose, and treat a particular disease, is the core of nuclear medicine [2]. The possibility of labeling the same agent with γ- or positron-emitting radionuclide well suited for imaging, as well as a α- or β-emitting nuclide suitable for therapy, makes nuclear medicine one the most appropriate discipline to exploit theranostics.

From the early experiences in 1940s and through the years, several theranostic approaches have been studied, performing a diagnostic molecular imaging followed by a personalized treatment decision based on the predictive value of the diagnostic scan.

1.1 Theranostics: Brief History

From an historical perspective, radioiodine was the first theranostic radiopharmaceutical in nuclear medicine, which was proposed for imaging and therapy in thyroid diseases.

In 1937, the first studies on radioactive iodine started, based on the known facts of thyroid physiology that indicated that iodine is selectively taken up by the thyroid gland and that in some measure gland's function is regulated by its iodine content. From this knowledge sprang the idea of potentially using "tagged" radioactive iodine as a physiologic indicator of thyroid functions [7]. Early experiments, by Hertz and Roberts, involved the administration of radioactive iodine (iodine-128) to rabbits. Their tissues were, then, collected and analyzed, in order to detect radioactive distribution with a Geiger-Müller counter. One rabbit, whose thyroid had been previously rendered hyperplastic through the injection of anterior pituitary extract (thyrotropin—TSH), showed particular iodine distribution: in none of the tissues or fluids examined were quantities of iodine found (exception made for the urinary tract), compared with that taken up by the thyroid. They, therefore, proved that the normal thyroid gland concentrated iodine and the hyperplastic gland took up even more, and, for the first time, hypothesized that their findings may be of therapeutic significance [7]. Researches proceeded and, in 1938, some longer-lasting radioisotopes of iodine were discovered:

iodine-126 (13 days half-life), iodine-130 (12.5 h half-life), and iodine-131 (8 days half-life), by Livingood and Seaborg and at the University of California, Berkeley [8].

Later on, two collaborators from Berkeley published the first data that showed how radio-iodine was taken up by the human thyroid, and that it could be detected in vivo: a realistic test for thyroid function was now in sight [9].

From late 1940, Hertz and Roberts used cyclo-tron's radioiodine to study more patients with Graves' hyperthyroidism. Soon they were able to calculate thyroid radioiodine uptake and moved on from the concept of "diagnostic tracer" to the intention to treat hyperthyroidism with radioac-tive iodine. In 1941 they started the adminis-tration with therapeutic purposes and the first reports, suggesting the use of radioactive iodine to cure hyperthyroidism of Graves' disease, were published on the Journal of the American Medical Association (JAMA) in May 1946 [10, 11]. The evidence was clear, the two published papers found the treatment successful and, only a month after, the Manhattan Project announced on the journal *Science* that radioactive iodine iso-topes were available for distribution on request for scientific purposes [12].

Shortly after, the first report of the use of radioactive iodine for the treatment of metastatic thyroid cancer was published by Seidlin et al. in 1948 [13]. Iodine-131 was administered to a patient who was clinically hyperthyroid despite having had a thyroidectomy for thyroid cancer. Pulmonary metastases were identified using a Geiger counter and the first rudimentary dosim-etry was performed. This report was followed by many case-reports that confirmed that meta-static thyroid cancer lesions could concentrate radioiodine.

Only with the benefit of hindsight, today, it is possible to acknowledge that these experiences represent the first applications of theranostics in molecular imaging and therapy, targeting the sodium-iodine symporter. Since then, the admin-istration of radiolabeled iodine for diagnostic imaging and therapy has represented an estab-lished and accepted theranostic approach in thy-roid diseases.

1.2 Theranostics: An Overview

For theranostic purposes, diverse combination of radiopharmaceuticals can be proposed: gamma- and beta-emitters radionuclides administered in different activities, different isotopes of the same element, different nuclides linked to the same carrier.

Nowadays, scintigraphy and radionuclide therapy with iodine-123/131 are used in the treat-ment and follow-up of patients with thyroid dis-eases, particularly differentiated thyroid cancer and hyperthyroidism. Gamma-camera can visu-alize accurate localization of sites of pathologi-cal radioiodine uptake, such as metastasis lesions or residual thyroid in patients with differentiated thyroid cancer who have undergone total thyroid-ectomy, because the lesions are highly efficient at trapping circulating iodine by expression of sodium-iodide symporter. Iodine-131 has been successfully used for the therapy of primary and metastatic lesions of differentiated thyroid cancer for many years. Scintigraphic scan using radio-active iodine can predict treatment efficacy, can potentially alter the decision to treat the patient, can finalize the subsequent therapeutic dose, and could be employed to perform dosimetric evalu-ation. Radioactive iodine dose selection is gener-ally based on patient risk factors. Since the release of radiation has high energy (364 keV γ-rays), whole body scintigraphy with ^{131}I has low spatial resolution and poor image quality [14].

Iodine-123, a lower 159 keV γ-emitter, has a higher counting rate compared to ^{131}I and pro-vides a higher lesion-to-background signal, so ^{123}I scanning offers excellent image quality compared to ^{131}I imaging, in thyroid carcinoma patients. Moreover, with the same administered activity, ^{123}I delivers an absorbed radiation dose that is approximately one-fifth that of ^{131}I, decreasing patients' radiation exposure. However, the clini-cal application of ^{123}I is limited by high cost due to accelerator production and report showed that diagnostic scans undervalue the disease burden compared to ^{131}I scans after treatment, especially in children and in other patients with prior radio-iodine therapy and/or distant metastasis. Few researches compared the diagnostic sensitivities of ^{123}I and ^{131}I whole-body imaging in differentiated thyroid cancer in thyroidectomized patients and found that ^{123}I appears adequate for imaging of residual thyroid tissue but is less sensitive than ^{131}I for imaging thyroid cancer metastases [14].

Iodine-124 (^{124}I) is a PET radiopharmaceutical with higher energy ($511, 603, 723, 1690$ keV) and a 4.2 days half-life, which potentially offers higher sensitivity and better imaging characteristics. Preliminary studies proved a high level of agreement between pre-therapeutic ^{124}I PET and post-therapeutic ^{131}I imaging in detecting iodine-positive thyroid cancer metastases. In addition, ^{124}I-PET proved to be a superior diagnostic tool in detecting residual, recurrent, and metastatic lesions with a higher sensitivity than the conventional ^{131}I scans. As an Auger electron emitter (9.2 per decay), there are potential therapeutic uses for this tracer, as well. Due to its cost and diagnostic reasons, ^{124}I PET/CT imaging is more common than ^{123}I scans but rarer than ^{131}I scans [14].

The role of radioactive iodine doesn't end with thyroid diseases. Iodine isotopes could be used to label different compound: a well-known example is represented by metaiodobenzylguanidine (mIBG).

mIBG is a guanethidine derivative developed in the late 1970s as diagnostic agent for imaging of adrenal medulla. It is an aralkylguanidine which is structurally similar to the neurotransmitter norepinephrine and is taken up by tumor originating from the neural crest. Since it is actively uptaken and stored in cytoplasmatic vesicles of tumor cells, whole-body imaging using radiolabeled mIBG has been used to stage, treat, and monitor therapy response in several endocrine tumors, since 1981 [15].

Iodine-123/131 mIBG scintigraphic scans are both well-established imaging modalities for diagnosis, staging, and restaging of tumors deriving from the neural crest. However, for clinical practice, the superiority of ^{123}I- over ^{131}I-labeled mIBG, for diagnostic purposes, has been ascertained. Indeed, for its physical properties, ^{123}I-allows to perform planar, whole-body and SPECT high-count scans, providing better spatial resolution than ^{131}I-mIBG, while delivering a lower radiation dose. The specificity in diagnosis has

remained above 95%, but sensitivity varies with the tumor nature: close to 90% for intra-adrenal pheochromocytomas but 70% or less for paragangliomas. Although diagnosis by radiolabeled mIBG has been supplemented and sometimes surpassed by newer scintigraphic agents, imaging with this radiopharmaceutical remains essential for optimal care of selected cases. The radiation delivered by high concentrations of ^{131}I-mIBG in malignant pheochromocytomas, paragangliomas, carcinoid tumors, and medullary thyroid carcinoma has reduced tumor volumes and lessened excretions of symptom-inflicting hormones, but its value as a therapeutic agent is being fulfilled primarily in treatment of neuroblastomas [16].

A well-established theranostic nuclides' pair is represented by Gallium-68 (^{68}Ga) and Lutetium-177 (^{177}Lu) or Yttrium-90 (^{90}Y). They are currently applied in the field of neuroendocrine tumors (NETs), replacing, despite its large use in the previous decade, Indium-111 (^{111}In).

NETs, in approximately 80% of the cases, overexpress somatostatin receptors (SSTRs) on cell surface, both in primary and in related metastasis. SSTRs presence allows theranostic application and targeting with peptide receptor radionuclide therapy (PRRT). PRRT consists in the systemic administration of a radiolabeled synthetic analog with a suitable beta-emitting radionuclide, which, once internalized through a specific receptor, irradiate tumor tissue. SSTRs have five subtypes termed SSTR1 to SSTR5, all of these receptors bind to natural somatostatin with high affinity. However, natural somatostatin exhibits a very short in vivo half-life of only 2–3 min; therefore, applications of natural somatostatin are limited. Considering these findings, various long-lived somatostatin analogs (SSAs) have been synthesized for medical imaging and therapy. Several radiolabeled SSAs have been proposed for PRRT and they are different in terms of radionuclide, somatostatin analog, and chelator [17].

The first nuclide applied to neuroendocrine tumors was ^{111}In. The physical properties of ^{111}In make it suitable for both diagnostic (γ-decay 245 keV and 171 keV) and therapeutic purposes (Auger electron emission). Auger electrons are high linear energy transfer particles, able to deliver high doses within a very short range (<10 μm). However, the high cytotoxic potential of the Auger electrons requires close proximity of the ^{111}In-labeled peptide within the nucleus, preferably intercalating with the DNA chain [17].

Indium-111 decay characteristics enable also dosimetric treatment planning. Dosimetry is facilitated by the γ-ray emission and the relatively long half-life (2.83 days), which matches the peptide biologic half-life. Therefore, a suitable number of scintigraphic images can be obtained over 3 days [17].

^{111}In-DTPA-octreotide, binding to SSTR2, was the first and most widely used radiopharmaceutical for detecting, staging and treat NETs. At diagnostic activity, its sensitivity is almost 80%, but its detection rate decreases with smaller lesions; at therapeutic activity, it has been employed with a good overall treatment effects [17, 18].

Despite its large use, in the previous decade, ^{111}In was abandoned and replaced by nuclides that guarantee a higher resolution in diagnostics, and good overall survival, improvement of quality of life, and less side effects in therapeutics.

Through the years, in the diagnostic field, several PET tracers have been proposed for functional imaging of NETs. Three [68]Ga- labeled somatostatin analogs are currently routinely used in clinical practice, thanks to their high affinity binding to SSTR2: ^{68}Ga-DOTA-D-Phe-Tyr3-octreotide (DOTATOC), ^{68}Ga-DOTA-1-Nal(3)-octreotide (DOTANOC), and ^{68}Ga-DOTA-D-Phe-Tyr3-octreotate (DOTATATE). Whereas in the therapeutic field, the most commonly used isotopes for treatment-intended radiolabeling of somatostatin analogs are the [90]Y (β-emitting isotope, Emax 2.28 MeV) or [177]Lu (decay β- 498 KeV, γ- 208 KeV) with DOTATOC or DOTATATE [13]. The recently published randomized Phase III NETTER-1 trial unequivocally demonstrated the efficacy of PRRT, using ^{177}Lu-DOTATATE, in patients with metastatic and progressive NETs with minimal side effects [19].

Specifically, in case of ^{177}Lu-peptide therapy, the isotope decay enables imaging, dosimetry, and therapy with the same compound. Whereas ^{111}In-octreotide was firstly proposed to depict

the dosimetry of ^{90}Y-peptides, but its use, suitable for diagnostics, is not recommended for dosimetric purposes, due to its different kinetics and receptor affinity properties [17]. Similarly, ^{68}Ga-peptides are striking diagnostics tracers but not suitable to simulate therapy, due to the short physical half-life (68 min) of ^{68}Ga as compared to the biological half-life of peptides, which impedes to derive the washout trend on the time-activity curves. Furthermore, it is not clear whether the ^{68}Ga properties might slightly alter the whole molecule behavior as compared to the therapeutic radiopharmaceuticals.

Labeled-SSAs diagnostic imaging and PRRT have been also applied in the diagnosis and treatment of recurrent meningiomas, malignant paragangliomas and pheochromocytomas and medullary thyroid cancers [18].

The success of the theranostic approach in the management of NETs with SSTRs targeting also prompted a case for exploring the possibility of targeting other peptide receptors. The expression of several bombesin receptor subtypes has been demonstrated in NETs, including the gastrin-releasing peptide (GRP) receptors. Particularly, the bombesin receptor antagonist demobesin showed superior in vivo stability, high tumor uptake and retention, and rapid pancreatic and renal clearance. The effective labeling and preclinical studies with GRP receptor antagonists has opened up a novel theranostic prospect in GRP receptor-positive tumors, including neuroendocrine tumors with [68]Ga-/^{177}Lu-labeled GRP receptor antagonists like demobesin [18].

Another application of the "theranostic couple" [68]Ga and ^{177}Lu can be found in the management of prostate cancer.

The prostate-specific membrane antigen (PSMA) is a transmembrane protein, upregulated in poorly differentiated, metastatic, and hormone-refractory prostate carcinomas, while physiological expression is restricted to only a few sites (such as the kidneys). In recent years, a number of PSMA-targeted nuclear imaging agents were developed [20, 21].

Thanks to its selective expression, PSMA targeting is of particular interest for the management in prostate cancer. Radiolabeled PSMA-617, a

1,4,7,10-tetraazacyclododecane-N,N',N'',N'''-tetraacetic acid (DOTA)-functionalized PSMA ligand, has been designed to enable a successful application for PET imaging (^{68}Ga) and radionuclide therapy (^{177}Lu) in clinical practice, revealing favorable kinetics with high tumor uptake and, consequently, opening the way towards a theranostic approach. Clinical studies performed so far demonstrated the promising potential of [68]Ga- and ^{177}Lu-labeled PSMA-617 in metastatic prostate cancer management [20, 21].

An ever-growing part of target therapy is represented by radiolabeled monoclonal antibodies (mAbs). Radioimmunoimaging has long been developed in parallel with radioimmunotherapy as a means for evaluating targeting and dosimetry of radiolabeled monoclonal antibodies. Technetium-99 m (^{99m}Tc), Copper-64 (^{64}Cu), ^{68}Ga, Yttrium-86 ([86]Y), Zirconium-89 ([89]Zr), ^{111}In, ^{123}I, [124]I, ^{131}I, and ^{177}Lu are the radionuclides most commonly used for molecular imaging with mAbs and antibody-related therapeutics. Selecting a suitable radionuclide generally starts by matching the serum half-life of the mAb or antibody-related therapeutic and the physical half-life of the radionuclide. This step is essential to minimize the time of exposure to radiation while ensuring that radioactivity to be detected long enough for the drug to bind the target [22].

In case of metal-based nuclides, such as ^{64}Cu, ^{68}Ga, [86]Y, [89]Zr, ^{111}In, and ^{177}Lu, a chelator is required. For human use, the chelator choice relies on the radionuclide, the stability of the chemical link, and the validation of clinical applicability. Analyzing the mAbs behavior, after binding the target, is of fundamental importance as well; radiometal-labeled drugs are metabolized and the nuclide is trapped intracellularly, thus guaranteeing a higher tumor-to-blood ratios. Whereas, iodine-labeled drugs are characterized by rapid renal clearance of the radionuclide from tumor cells [22].

A well-known application of radioimmunotherapy is the Food and Drug Administration-approved agent Zevalin (Spectrum Pharmaceuticals, Inc., Henderson, NV). Zevalin is labeled with pure beta-emitter therapeutic isotope ^{90}Y that provides no imaging emission.

However [86]Y, a positron emitter yttrium isotope, could be a good choice as a surrogate pre-therapy PET isotopically matched surrogate for ^{90}Y radiation doses estimations [23].

In recent years, molecular imaging using the positron emitter [89]Zr for antibody labeling has increased. Zirconium-89 physical half-life (78.4 h) generally matches the serum half-life of most mAbs and antibody-related therapeutics in vivo, thus achieving high tumor-to-background ratios, and it allows a stable link with mAbs and antibody-related therapeutics (such as [89]Zr-labeled trastuzumab and cetuximab) [22].

Copper-64 is a useful and practical theranostic radionuclide. It enables both PET-imaging and radionuclide therapy, because it is characterized by β+ decay (0.653 MeV, 17.4%), β− decay (0.574 MeV, 40%), and electron capture (42.6%). The photons generated from electron–positron annihilation can be detected by PET, and the β− particles and Auger electrons emitted from this nuclide can damage tumor cells' DNA. Clinical PET studies using ^{64}Cu-labeled agents, such as ^{64}Cu-diacetyl-bis (N4-methylthiosemicarbazone) (^{64}Cu-ATSM) and ^{64}Cu-labeled trastuzumab, have shown the utility of [64]Cu- for imaging in humans. Data from many preclinical studies have also demonstrated the therapeutic effectiveness of ^{64}Cu-labeled agents, such as ^{64}Cu-ATSM, ^{64}Cu-labeled Arg-Gly-Asp peptide, and ^{64}Cu-labeled antibodies. Recently, a first-in-human study of radionuclide therapy with [64]CuCl2 was conducted in Europe, and it was reported that the patient showed a remarkable reduction of tumor volume without side effects, supporting the applicability of ^{64}Cu in clinical use for therapy [24].

An *unconventional* theranostic application can be found in the use of labeled microspheres for selective hepatic treatment. Radioembolization is an interventional oncologic treatment during which radioactive microspheres are administered in hepatic arterial vessels supplying the liver and its tumors. [166]Ho-poly(l-lactic acid) microspheres have been developed as an alternative to ^{90}Y-microspheres specifically to enable the in vivo visualization of microspheres biodistribution after radioembolization. The physical properties of ^{166}Ho- (β- decay Emax 1.85 MeV, γ- decay Emax = 0.081 MeV) enable SPECT and MRI imaging. They may, therefore, represent a step forward from ^{90}Y-microspheres, allowing not only post-therapy imaging but also theranostic application. Even though a scintigraphic scan, acquired after the administration of ^{166}Ho-microspheres at "tracer activity," is not properly a diagnostic tool per se, it still has a predictive intent on treatment outcome and could also enable dosimetric purposes, in order to design a personalized treatment planning, on the base of tumor and healthy liver doses [24].

A mention aside from radionuclide therapy should be made. In recent years, a ^{99m}Tc-labeled chemotherapy analog has been developed which can be used for the selection of patients with tumors expressing folate receptors, enabling the selection of those patients who will benefit from chemotherapy with folate receptor-targeted agents while sparing those patients who do not express this receptor a potentially toxic but probably ineffective course of treatment [2].

The above is just a small selection of an ever-growing number of examples which clearly illustrate that nuclear medicine has had both a rich history and an evolving role in theranostics, contributing to the birth of the concept itself, applying it and modernizing it, as time passed by, therefore contributing to the development of personalized medicine.

1.3 Theranostics: Critical Analysis and Future Perspectives

Theranostics is currently applied in clinical management on a daily basis. It is, therefore, important to have a comprehensive look at both advantages and disadvantages of this strategy.

Ideally, for theranostic use, the radiopharmaceutical employed should be constituted with the same dual-purpose radionuclide, with both imaging and therapeutic emissions. In this first-case scenario, even though using the same nuclide, the administration of high-dose radiopharmaceutical, for therapeutic purposes, might impair

the reproducibility of what previously diagnosed with low-dose.

In the second best situation, a radionuclide pair (imaging photon emitter, either gamma or positron, and a counterpart therapeutic particle emitter, with the same electronic structure) can be used as well. Although many theranostic imaging/therapy radionuclide pairs may have the same electronic structure, their production and processing methodologies may be significantly different. Consequently, their chemistry and in vivo behavior may be different as well, because of differences in chemical species, charge, specific activity, and/or the amount of chemical and radionuclidic chemical impurities, which cannot be totally removed [4]. An example can be found in the fact that, even when using the same chelator, the chemical properties of ^{68}Ga- and ^{177}Lu-labeled compounds are not identical due to the different coordination chemistry of these radiometals, which may result in different in vivo kinetics [21].

Another issue, that has to be dealt with, is the fact that half-life of the imaging PET nuclide, in most cases, might be much shorter than the usually (desirable) longer half-life of the therapeutic nuclide. In most situations, the determination of longer-term biodistribution would be crucial for dosimetry, but this information would not be achievable using the shorter-lived positron-emitter for pretherapy imaging.

A sore point to deal with is the limited resources for establishing the evidence base that usually accompanies registration and approval of cancer therapies. There has been a lack of randomized controlled trial data comparing radionuclide therapies with other forms of therapy and virtually none testing the integrated theranostic approach. Aside from randomized NETTER-1 clinical trial, whose preliminary results showed the potentiality of PRRT at the 2016 Gastrointestinal Cancers Symposium, there is a strong need of further, randomized, controlled experiences, in order to gain deserved visibility in clinician world [19].

On the other hand, nuclear medicine has gained more than 80 years of experience in theranostics. From thyroid cancer management with radioiodine and forth, it is possible to obtain some key points to properly apply targeted medicine and theranostics principles and enhance their advantages.

An optimal patient selection is crucial, based on the knowledge that target expression is not the only aspect to take into account. Several prognostic factors influence therapy outcome, such as tumor burden, disease localization, and presence of heterogenous disease with subclones of tumor cells lacking target expression.

The possibility of associating cytostatic treatments before, between, and after radionuclide therapy should not be underestimated (i.e., "cold" somatostatin analogs during PRRT in NETs treatment; thyrotropin suppression with supra-physiologic thyroid hormone replacement administration in thyroid cancer after radioiodine treatment).

Another well-established procedure is the pharmacological increase of radiosensitivity in order to enhance therapy effectiveness (i.e., capecitabine or capecitabine and temozolomide or 5-fluorouracil in NETs before and during PRRT [25, 26]; induction of upregulation of iodine transporter expression through increased thyrotropin levels, endogenous or exogenous, in thyroid cancer before radioiodine treatment).

Prospective dosimetry is a promising aspect of theranostics, not widely applied due to procedures execution limitations, but yet appealing.

A feature entailed in the concept of theranostics, as much as therapeutics and diagnostics, is prognostics. Many diagnostic tests in nuclear medicine are associated with a clear prognostic stratification. For instance, after radioiodine treatment in thyroid cancer, a negative diagnostic whole-body ^{131}I scintigraphy, combined with clinical elements, establishes that ^{131}I therapy is no longer necessary and is clearly associated with a lower risk of tumor recurrence, as well.

Holding a wide and depth knowledge of advantages and disadvantages that ensue from the application of theranostics is an essential requirement to properly exploit this tool in clinical management. Conscious of its limits, theranostics can be successfully applied as a powerful strategy in cancer treatment, and nuclear medicine owns the tools to play a central role in this field.

References

1. Del Vecchio S, Zannetti A, Fonti R, Pace L, Salvatore M. Nuclear imaging in cancer theranostics. Q J Nucl Med Mol Imaging. 2007;51(2):152–63.
2. Verburg FA, Heinzel A, Hänscheid H, Mottaghy FM, Luster M, Giovanella L. Nothing new under the nuclear sun: towards 80 years of theranostics in nuclear medicine. Eur J Nucl Med Mol Imaging. 2014;41(2):199–201.
3. De Nardo GL, De Nardo SJ. Concepts, consequences and implications of theranosis. Semin Nucl Med. 2012;42(3):147–50.
4. Srivastava SC. Paving the way to personalized medicine: production of some promising theragnostic radionuclides at Brookhaven national laboratory. Semin Nucl Med. 2012;42:151–63.
5. Taïeb D, Hicks RJ, Pacak K. Nuclear medicine in cancer theranostics: beyond the target. J Nucl Med. 2016;57(11):1659–60.
6. Dagogo-Jack I, Shaw AT. Tumor heterogeneity and resistance to cancer therapies. Nat Rev Clin Oncol. 2018;15(2):81–94.
7. Hertz S, Roberts A, Evans RD. Radioactive iodine as an indicator in the study of thyroid physiology. Exp Biol Med. 1938;38(4):510–3.
8. Livingood JJ, Seaborg GT. Radioactive isotopes of iodine. Phys Rev. 1938;53:775.
9. Perlman I, Chaikoff IL, Morton ME. Radioactive Iodine as an indicator of the metabolism of iodine I. The turnover of iodine in the tissue of the normal animal, with particular reference to the thyroid. J Biol Chem. 1941;139:433.
10. Hertz S, Robert A. Radioactive iodine in the study of thyroid physiology VII. The use of radioactive iodine therapy in hyperthyroidism. JAMA. 1946;131:81.
11. Chapman EM, Evans RD. The treatment of hyperthyroidism with the radioactive iodine. JAMA. 1946;131:86.
12. Pollard WG. Availability of radioactive isotopes. Science. 1946;103:697.
13. Seidlin SM, Oshry E, Yalow AA. Spontaneous and experimentally induced uptake of radioactive iodine in metastases from thyroid carcinoma; a preliminary report. J Clin Endocrinol Metab. 1948;8(6):423–32.
14. Liu H, Wang X, Yang R, Zeng W, Peng D, Li J, Wang H. Recent development of nuclear molecular imaging in thyroid cancer. Biomed Res Int. 2018;2018:2149532.
15. Naranjo A, Parisi MT, Shulkin BL, London WB, Matthay KK, Kreissman SG, Yanik GA. Comparison of 123I-metaiodobenzylguanidine (MIBG) and 131I-MIBG semi-quantitative scores in predicting survival in patients with stage 4 neuroblastoma: a report from the children's oncology group. Pediatr Blood Cancer. 2011;56(7):1041–5.
16. Sisson JC, Yanik GA. Theranostics: evolution of the radiopharmaceutical meta-iodobenzylguanidine in endocrine tumors. Semin Nucl Med. 2012;42(3):171–84.

17. Werner RA, Bluemel C, Allen-Auerbach MS, Higuchi T. Herrmann K. 68Gallium- and 90Yttrium-/177Lutetium: "theranostic twins" for diagnosis and treatment of NETs. Ann Nucl Med. 2015;29:1–7.
18. Baum RP, Kulkarni HR, Carreras C. Peptides and receptors in image-guided therapy: theranostics for neuroendocrine neoplasms. Semin Nucl Med. 2012;42(3):190–207.
19. Strosberg J, El-Haddad G, Wolin E, Hendifar A, Yao J, Chasen B, Mittra E, Kunz PL, Kulke MH, Jacene H, Bushnell D, O'Dorisio TM, Baum RP, Kulkarni HR, Caplin M, Lebtahi R, Hobday T, Delpassand E, Van Cutsem E, Benson A, Srirajaskanthan R, Pavel M, Mora J, Berlin J, Grande E, Reed N, Seregni E, Öberg K, Lopera Sierra M, Santoro P, Thevenet T, Erion JL, Ruszniewski P, Kwekkeboom D, Krenning E, NETTER-1 Trial Investigators. Phase 3 trial of 177Lu-dotatate for midgut neuroendocrine tumors. N Engl J Med. 2017;376(2):125–35.
20. Afshar-Oromieh A, Hetzheim H, Kratochwil C, Benesova M, Eder M, Neels OC, Eisenhut M, Kübler W, Holland-Letz T, Giesel FL, Mier W, Kopka K, Haberkorn U. The theranostic PSMA ligand PSMA-617 in the diagnosis of prostate cancer by PET/CT: biodistribution in humans, radiation dosimetry, and first evaluation of tumor lesions. J Nucl Med. 2015;56(11):1697–705.
21. Umbricht CA, Benesova M, Schmid RM, Turler A, Schibli R, van der Meulen NP, Muller C. 44Sc-PSMA-617 for radiotheragnostics in tandem with 177Lu-PSMA-617-preclinical investigations in comparison with 68Ga-PSMA-11 and 68Ga-PSMA-617. EJNMMI Res. 2017;7(1):9.
22. Moek KL, Giesen D, Kok IC, de Groot DJA, Jalving M, Fehrmann RSN, Lub-de Hooge MN, Brouwers AH, de Vries EGE. Theranostics using antibodies and antibody-related therapeutics. J Nucl Med. 2017;58:83S–90S.
23. Nayak TK, Brechbiel MW. 86Y based PET radiopharmaceuticals: radiochemistry and biological applications. Med Chem. 2011;7(5):380–8.
24. Yoshii Y, Yoshimoto M, Matsumoto H, Tashima H, Iwao Y, Takuwa H, Yoshida E, Wakizaka H, Yamaya T, Zhang MR, Sugyo A, Hanadate S, Tsuji AB, Higashi T. Integrated treatment using intraperitoneal radioimmunotherapy and positron emission tomography-guided surgery with 64Cu-labeled cetuximab to treat early- and late-phase peritoneal dissemination in human gastrointestinal cancer xenografts. Oncotarget. 2018;9(48):28935–50.
25. Claringbold PG, Brayshaw PA, Price RA, Turner JH. Phase II study of radiopeptide 177Lu-octreotate and capecitabine therapy of progressive disseminated neuroendocrine tumors. Eur J Nucl Med Mol Imaging. 2011;38(2):302–11.
26. Thakral P, Sen I, Pant V, Gupta SK, Dureja S, Kumari J, Kumar S, Un P, Malasani V. Dosimetric analysis of patients with gastro entero pancreatic neuroendocrine tumors (NETs) treated with PRCRT (peptide receptor chemo radionuclide therapy) using Lu-177 DOTATATE and capecitabine/temozolomide (CAP/TEM). Br J Radiol. 2018;91:20170172.

Radioiodine Therapy of Benign Thyroid Diseases

2

Alfredo Campennì, Desiree Deandreis,
Monica Finessi, Rosaria Maddalena Ruggeri,
and Sergio Baldari

2.1 Hyperthyroidism: Definition and Epidemiology

Thyrotoxicosis represents a clinical condition that results from excess thyroid hormone(s) levels and action in peripheral tissues, either with or without increased synthesis of thyroid hormone(s) by the gland. It has multiple different etiologies and potential therapies; therefore, an accurate diagnosis is mandatory for appropriate treatment [1]. In general, thyrotoxicosis can be the consequence of (1) active production of excess thyroid hormone(s) by the thyroid or (2) passive release of stored hormone(s) in the bloodstream because of gland inflammation or mechanical insult. More rarely, thyrotoxicosis can occur as the consequence of exposure to either endogenous or exogenous extra-thyroidal sources of thyroid hormone(s) (Table 2.1) [1]. Hyperthyroidism is a form of thyrotoxicosis due to excessive synthesis and secretion of thyroid hormone(s) by the thyroid [1]. It is generally defined as overt or subclinical, depending on the severity of biochemical abnormalities. Overt hyperthyroidism is defined as a low (usually undetectable) serum thyrotropin (TSH) with elevated serum levels of triiodothyronine (T3) and/or free thyroxine (free T4). By contrast, subclinical hyperthyroidism is defined as serum free T4 (FT4) and total or free T3 (FT3) levels within their respective reference ranges in the presence of abnormal serum TSH, and it is further subdivided into a mild (low TSH, <0.4 mU/mL) and severe (undetectable TSH <0.01 mU/mL) form [1, 2]. Both overt and subclinical disease may lead to characteristic signs and symptoms, although subclinical hyperthyroidism is usually considered milder [2, 3].

The overall prevalence of hyperthyroidism is estimated to be ∼2–3% in women and 0.2–0.5% in men. Incidence is highest in Caucasians and in iodine-deficient areas and rises with age [4–6]. The main causes of hyperthyroidism include Graves' disease (GD), toxic adenoma (TA), and toxic multinodular goiter (TMNG). GD accounts for ∼80% of cases in iodine-sufficient areas and is more prevalent among smokers, whereas autonomously functioning thyroid nodules (either TMNG or TA) are more common than GD in iodine-deficient areas, especially in older patients [1, 4, 7, 8].

A. Campennì (✉) · S. Baldari
Department of Biomedical and Dental Sciences and Morpho-Functional Imaging, Nuclear Medicine Unit, University of Messina, Messina, Italy
e-mail: acampenni@unime.it; sbaldari@unime.it

D. Deandreis · M. Finessi
Department of Medical Sciences, Nuclear Medicine Unit, University of Turin, Turin, Italy
e-mail: desiree.deandreis@unito.it

R. M. Ruggeri
Department of Clinical and Experimental Medicine, Unit of Endocrinology, University of Messina, Messina, Italy
e-mail: rmruggeri@unime.it

© Springer Nature Switzerland AG 2019
L. Giovanella (ed.), *Nuclear Medicine Therapy*, https://doi.org/10.1007/978-3-030-17494-1_2

Table 2.1 Multiple etiologies, different mechanism, and main diagnostic features of thyrotoxicosis

	Etio-pathogenetic mechanism	Diagnostic features
Thyrotoxicosis with hyperthyroidism		
Graves' disease	Thyrotropin receptor antibodies (TRAb) stimulate the TSH-R	Diffuse goiter. Orbitopathy may be present. Increased RAIU and diffuse radioisotope uptake on thyroid scan. Positive TRAb and TPO-Ab
Toxic adenoma	Monoclonal autonomously functional benign lesion. Activating mutations in TSH receptor or G proteins	Increased or normal RAIU; radioisotope focal uptake in the nodule with suppressed uptake in the surrounding thyroid tissue on scan; TPO-Ab and TRAb absent
Toxic multinodular goiter	Functional autonomy within multiple monoclonal benign lesions. Activating mutations in TSH-R receptor or G proteins	Increased or normal RAIU; multiple focal areas of increased and reduced uptake on scan; TPO-Ab and TRAb absent
Familial congenital hyperthyroidism	Activating mutations in TSH-R ß or G proteins	Diffuse goiter. Increased RAIU and diffuse radiotracer uptake on thyroid scan. TRAb and TPO-Ab absent.
TSH secreting pituitary adenoma	Pituitary adenoma	Raised serum TSH and α-subunit with raised peripheral serum thyroid hormones
Pituitary resistance to thyroid hormone	Mutation of T3 receptor β THRB	Raised or normal serum TSH with raised peripheral serum thyroid hormones
Gestational thyrotoxicosis	Stimulation of TSH-R by human chorionic gonadotropin	First trimester; often in the setting of hyperemesis or multiple gestation.
Choriocarcinoma/ Molar pregnancy	Stimulation of TSH-R by human chorionic gonadotropin	Molar pregnancy
Drug-induced hyperthyroidism (checkpoint inhibitors, interferon alfa,…)	Induction of thyroid autoimmunity (Graves' disease)	Increased RAIU and diffuse radioisotope uptake on thyroid scan. Positive TRAb and/or TPO-Ab
Iodine or iodine-containing drugs (amiodarone-induce thyrotoxicosis type 1)	Jod-Basedow phenomenon; excess iodine results in unregulated thyroid hormone production	Low to undetectable RAIU
Thyrotoxicosis without hyperthyroidism		
Painless, postpartum and/or sporadic thyroiditis	Autoimmune, release of stored thyroid hormones	Low to undetectable RAIU and radioisotope uptake on thyroid scan; TPO-Ab present. Postpartum form occurs within 12 months after pregnancy
Subacute (granulomatous, de Quervain's) thyroiditis	Viral; thyroid inflammation with release of stored thyroid hormone	Neck pain. Low to undetectable RAIU and radioisotope uptake on thyroid scan; low or absent TPO-Ab
Acute infectious thyroiditis	Bacterial or fungal thyroid infection; release of stored thyroid hormones	Neck pain. Low to undetectable and RAIU and radioisotope uptake on thyroid scan
Iatrogenic thyrotoxicosis (drugs, such as lithium, interferon alfa, checkpoint inhibitors; radiation…) Amiodarone-induced thyrotoxicosis type II	Inflammatory thyroiditis with destruction of thyroid follicles and release of stored hormones	Low to and low radioisotope uptake on thyroid scan and radioisotope uptake on thyroid scan; low or absent TPO-Ab
Extra-thyroidal sources of thyroid hormone		
Struma ovarii	Functional autonomy within an ovarian teratoma with differentiation into thyroid cells	Low to undetectable RAIU and radioisotope uptake on thyroid scan; raised uptake in the pelvis
Widely metastatic functional follicular thyroid carcinoma	Thyroid hormone production by large tumor masses with foci of functional autonomy	Differentiated thyroid carcinoma with bulky metastases; tumor radioactive iodine uptake on whole-body scan.
Exogenous thyroid hormone (thyrotoxicosis factitia)	Iatrogenic or factitious excess ingestion of thyroid hormone	Low to undetectable RAIU and radioisotope uptake on thyroid scan; low or absent TPO-Ab

TSH Thyrotropin, *TSH-R* Thyrotropin receptor, *TRAb* Thyrotropin receptor antibodies, *TPO-Ab* Thyroperoxidase antibodies, *RAIU* radioiodine uptake

2.1.1 Graves' Disease

Graves' disease (GD) represents the most common cause of persistent hyperthyroidism in adults from iodine-sufficient areas, with an incidence peak between 30 and 50 years of age and a higher prevalence in women (1:5–7) [7–10]. Its annual incidence is estimated to be 20–50 cases per 100,000 individuals/year [8, 10].

GD is autoimmune in etiology and is due to the loss of immune tolerance to thyroid self-antigens with production of organ-specific autoantibodies that specifically target the gland [8, 10]. In particular, GD is associated with a humoral response against the TSH receptor (TRH-R): autoantibodies against TRH-R, the so-called TRAb, promote thyroid growth and function via TRH-R activation, leading to hyperthyroidism and goiter [8, 10].

Additional peripheral manifestations include Graves' orbitopathy (GO), acropachy, and pretibial mixedema, which can vary greatly in frequency and intensity. The cause of peripheral tissue involvement is less clear. Given the presence of THSR in orbital and skin fibroblasts, these organs might be targeted by TRAb [3, 11]. Underlying these processes there is a complex interplay between genetic and environmental factors: such an organ-specific autoimmune disease develops in genetically susceptible individuals triggered by several different environmental and existential factors [8, 10]. Patients often have a family history or past medical history of other autoimmune diseases (e.g., rheumatoid arthritis, vitiligo, pernicious anemia, celiac disease) [12–14].

2.1.2 Toxic Nodular Disease (TA and TMNG)

Autonomously functioning thyroid nodules—either isolated or in the context of a multinodular goiter—are a relatively common finding in iodine-deficient areas, when they largely outnumber GD as the leading cause of hyperthyroidism, mostly in elderly [2, 15–17]. Somatic activating mutations of the thyrotropin receptor (TSHR)

gene and the gene encoding the α subunit of the stimulatory GTP-binding protein (Gsα) represent the main cause of TA [18]. TMNGs typically occur in patients who have had a known history of nontoxic goiter for many years or decades. Such patients experience a progressive increase in size and number of nodules, resulting from chronic TSH stimulation in response to low iodine intake, and may develop autonomous growth and function over time. Somatic mutations of TSHR and/or Gsα gene have also been described in many—but not all—TMNG, as well as in TA, accounting for development of autonomy [18–20].

2.1.3 Natural History and Clinical Features

Presentation is mainly related to the severity and duration of hyperthyroidism, with a variable expression [2, 3, 8–10].

GD is typically characterized by sudden appearance of hyperthyroidism, mostly overt form, and diffuse goiter. By contrast, nodular autonomy (either due to TA or TMNG) progress gradually from subclinical to overt hyperthyroidism over the years, and it is quite common that administration of pharmacologic amounts of iodine (e.g., amiodarone, iodinated contrast) may trigger overt hyperthyroidism in such patients. Remission is rare in nodular autonomy, which is usually progressive, while it can occur in up to 30% of GD, especially in mild forms [4, 8, 9].

Clinical manifestations include local symptoms (i.e., dysphagia, dysphonia, or dyspnea), usually in individuals with large goiters, and systemic manifestations related to hyperthyroidism [3, 8] (Table 2.2). Given the broad action of thyroid hormones on most organs and tissues, the signs and symptoms of hyperthyroidism are numerous and greatly variable also in relation to patient' age and underlying comorbidities (Table 2.2). Younger patients tend to exhibit symptoms of sympathetic activation, such as anxiety, hyperactivity, heat intolerance, and tremor, while older patients present more frequently with unexplained weight loss and cardiovascular symptoms/signs [8, 21]. Atrial fibrillation can

Table 2.2 Clinical features of Graves' disease and autonomously functioning thyroid nodule(s)

	Signs	Symptoms
Systemic manifestations related to hyperthyroidism	Tremor, hyperkinesis, hyperreflexia Tachycardia (50%), atrial fibrillation (>10% of ≥60-year-old patients), systolic hypertension, cardiac failure Wet/warm skin, palmar erythema and onycolysis Weight loss, muscular hypotrophy Dermopathy (pretibial myxoedema) Acropachy *rare: thyroid storm*	Palpitations Increased perspiration, heat intolerance, fatigue, muscle weakness, increased appetite, weight loss Thirst and polyuria Pruritus Menstrual disturbances in women (oligo- or amenorrhea), loss of libido Diarrhea Anxiety, altered mood, nervousness Apathy, lethargy (*apathetic thyrotoxicosis*, in the elderly)
Local manifestations related to large goiter	Palpable/enlarged thyroid and/or nodules	Mechanical symptoms (dysphagia, dyspnea, dysphonia)
Graves' Orbitopathy (GO)	*Soft tissues involvement* Palpebral swelling/erythema, caruncle swelling, conjunctivae hyperemia, chemosis Eyelid lag, retraction, or both Proptosis (exophthalmos) Corneal involvement (exposure keratitis) Extraocular muscles involvement (movement limitations) Optical nerve involvement (up to *dysthyroid optic neuropathy, DON*)	Increased lacrimation Foreign body sensation Photophobia Ocular pain (spontaneous/at gaze), Diplopia Blurred vision, reduced visual acuity

occur in more than 10% of 60-year-old individuals or older, and it can be the first and only manifestation in elderly [21–23]. Increasing age, male sex, and underlying cardiovascular disease are risk factors for atrial fibrillation, an independent predictor of mortality [2, 22].

Clinical presentation of GD is also characterized by the peculiar involvement of peripheral tissues [3, 8–11]. GO, the most common and serious extra-thyroidal manifestation, affects up to 50% of GD patients [8, 11]. GO usually appears together with the thyroid affection or slowly after its onset [11]. It comprehends various degrees of exophthalmos, soft tissue inflammation, and muscular impairment and it threatens sight as a consequence of corneal breakdown or optic neuropathy in 3–5% of affected patients (Table 2.2) [11].

2.1.4 Diagnosis and Treatment

Apart from a detailed personal and familiar history and an accurate clinical examination, the diagnosis of hyperthyroidism relies on the bio-chemical appearance of hyperthyroidism, overt or even subclinical (low TSH with high or normal levels of FT3 and FT4, respectively). FT3/FT4 ratio is generally increased. A T3 toxicosis (low/suppressed TSH with high FT3 and normal FT4) may represent the earliest stage of hyperthyroidism, mainly due to TMNG and/or TA. Serum antithyroid antibodies (anti-thyroperoxidase or TPO Ab, and anti-thyroglobulin or Tg-Ab) are usually absent in autonomously functioning thyroid nodules, while present in GD. Positivity of TRAb (99% sensitivity and specificity) represents the diagnostic hallmark of GD. However, TRAb may decline and may not be detectable in very mild GD or if measured after antithyroid drugs have been commenced [1, 4, 8, 10]. If TRAb is negative end/or the diagnosis is unclear, 131-radioiodine uptake (RAIU) and thyroid scintigraphy with either 123-radioiodine or ^{99m}Tc-pertechnetate are indicated. First of all, RAIU allows distinguishing causes of thyrotoxicosis with elevated or normal uptake over the thyroid gland (hyperthyroidism) from those with near-absent uptake (thyrotoxicosis without hyperthyroidism) [1] (Table 2.1). RAIU is usually elevated in patients with GD and normal or high in toxic nodular disease, while it is very low or absent in painless, postpartum, or subacute thyroiditis, factitious ingestion of thyroid hormone or iodine-induced thyrotoxicosis. Thyroid scintigraphy reveals an increased and diffuse uptake in both lobes in GD, and a focal uptake in TA with suppressed uptake in the surrounding and contralateral thyroid tissue. In TMNG the scintiscan demonstrates one or more "hot" nodules alternating with areas of reduced/suppressed uptake [1, 4, 8]. However, coexistent nontoxic nodules or fibrosis in GD, large areas of autonomy in TMNG or interfering factors (i.e., administration of iodinated contrast in the preceding 1–6 months) make hard the diagnosis on the sole basis of radionuclide uptake. Thyroid ultrasonography represents a useful tool in differential diagnosis of thyrotoxicosis. In GD, thyroid US demonstrates an enlarged, hypoecoic gland, with or without nodules, with an important increase of vascularization at color flow Doppler evaluation. Doppler flow evaluation can be helpful in distinguishing between GD and destructive thyroiditis, particularly when radionuclide administration is contraindicated, such as during pregnancy and lactation [1, 4]. In TA and mostly in TMNG, autonomously functioning thyroid nodules can be exactly identified by matching thyroid US and scintigraphy. Also US provide useful information concerning nodule's size and ecographic features.

The treatment of hyperthyroidism is aimed to restore euthyroidism and is based on either medical treatment with antithyroid drugs (titration or block and replace regimen) able to block the excessive thyroid hormone production, or on ablation/reduction of thyroid mass using surgery or radioactive iodine [1]. Antithyroid drugs (the thionamides, carbimazole, methimazole, and propylthiouracil) can be used as a first-line treatment in GD, since they achieve long-term remission in approximately 30% of cases. They can also be used as a pretreatment in selected patients prior to radioactive iodine therapy or prior to surgery. Beta-adrenergic blockade is recommended in patients with symptomatic thyrotoxicosis,

especially in elderly patients and those with cardiovascular disease [1].

2.2 Radioactive Iodine Therapy (RAIT) in Hyperthyroid Patients

In 2016, the nuclear medicine community celebrated the first 75 years of 131-radioiodine use to cure patients in hyperthyroid status. It was a fundamental step back then in the management of hyperthyroid patients since, for the first time, the toxic thyroid disease [diffuse or (multi)-nodular] could definitively be treated without the need of using a surgical approach, thus drastically reducing both side effects due to surgery (e.g., nerve palsy, hypoparathyroidism, hemorrhage) and healthcare costs.

From its first use, millions of people have been treated, worldwide. The rationale underlying nuclear medicine therapy is the ability of follicular thyroid cells to uptake 131-radioiodine (like iodine absorbed in the diet).

Today, 131-radioiodine represents the first example of "theranostic" radiotracer: its (−ve)-beta electrons allow us to obtain the therapeutic effect, while gamma-emission shows its distribution in the gland.

131-Radioiodine therapy has two main aims: the first is to correct hyperthyroidism reaching a euthyroid state as soon as possible (the optimal result for patients affected by (multi)-nodular toxic disease) or a hypothyroid state (the optimal result for patients with diffuse toxic disease); the second is to reduce whole gland or toxic (multi)-nodular volume.

2.2.1 Patients Preparation for Radioiodine Therapy

Specific antithyroid drugs (ATD) [i.e., methimazole (MMI), carbimazolo, or propylthiouracil (PTU)] such as Levo-Thyroxine, and iodine-containing products (e.g., toothpaste, disinfectant, hair dye) should be discontinued or avoided before radioactive iodine therapy (RAIT) as they can reduce radioiodine thyroid uptake thus reducing the success rate of the treatment. Should a patient be undergoing amiodarone therapy, RAIT must be postponed for at least six months after the last amiodarone administration. However, in these patients it is obligatory to evaluate radioiodine thyroid uptake (RAIU) before RAIT [1, 24].

Similarly, RAIT must be postponed in patients who have undergone radiographic studies with contrast agent administration (i.e., computed tomography (CT), from several weeks to many months after, taking into account contrast agent type (i.e., lipophilic or water soluble) [25, 26]. A special diet is not required before RAIT. However, some food types (e.g., fish, eggs, and milk), nutritional supplements, seaweeds, and iodine salt should be reduced or avoided for at least 7 days before RAIT, mainly in patients with low radioiodine uptake values. In patients whose diet is mainly based on seaweed or is rich in supplements containing iodide, an iodine urine measurement should be performed before RAIT [1] (Table 2.3). In young female patients who could

Table 2.3 Thyroid drugs, medications, and iodide-containing supplements that can reduce radioiodine thyroid uptake

Type of medication	Recommended time of withdrawal
Water-soluble intravenous radiographic contrast agents	6–8 wk[a], assuming normal renal function
Lipophilic intravenous radiographic contrast agents	1–6 mo[b]
Thyroxine	3–4 wk
Triiodothyronine	10–14 d[c]
Antithyroid drugs (methimazole, carbimazolo, propylthiouracil)	5–7 d
Nutrition supplements containing iodide	7–10 d
Kelp, agar, carrageenan, Lugol solution	2–3 wk., depending on iodide content
Saturated solution of potassium iodide	2–3 wk.
Topical iodine (e.g., surgical skin preparation)	2–3 wk.
Amiodarone	3–6 mo or longer

[a]wk = weeks
[b]mo = months
[c]d = days

be pregnant, a blood test must be performed within 72 h before RAIT since pregnancy is an absolute contraindication for RAIT. A pregnancy test is not necessary in female patients with documented hysterectomy/ovariectomy or tubal ligation. Finally, pregnancy must be avoided for six months after RAIT [25, 27].

Breastfeeding must be interrupted: RAIT should not be performed before 6 weeks after breastfeeding withdrawal to avoid high radioiodine uptake in hypertrophied breast, thus lowering the absorbed radiation dose [1, 25, 28].

2.2.2 Diffuse Toxic Goiter (Graves' Disease—GD)

RAIT is a safe, effective therapeutic option for GD patients [29].

GD patients may undergo RAIT as a first option care if: (1) they are >10 years, any gender, and have small to medium goiter and inactive Graves' orbitopathy (GO); (2) they are >10 years, any gender, and have small to medium goiter and low to mild active GO (using glucocorticoid therapy in patients with higher risk features, like smokers); (3) they have comorbidities increasing surgical risk (i.e., heart failure, pulmonary hypertension, systemic hypertension refractory to drugs, laryngeal nerve palsy); (4) there are contraindications to ATD (or patients with already documented adverse reaction); (5) there is recurrent disease after surgical therapy; (6) they are elderly with comorbidities (in particular metabolic comorbidities); (7) access to a high volume thyroid surgeon (mainly if children) is limited or not possible [1, 30].

On the contrary, RAIT is not administered in GD patients: (1) who are pregnant; (2) with the (multi)-nodular variant of GD with suspected or confirmed thyroid cancer; (3) with very large goiter; (4) with active GO of moderate to severe degree and high TRAb levels (mainly if smokers); (5) who are ≤5 years [1, 30–35].

RAIT should be delayed as much as possible in children between 5 and 10 years of age. In any case, in the pediatric setting, RAI administered activity should not be higher than 370 MBq [1].

The first aim of RAIT is to change the clinical status of patients from hyperthyroid to hypothyroid according to the current *"ablative dose concept"* based on evidence that the definitive success rate is much higher than that obtained according to the previous *"function oriented concept"* (>90% vs. < 70%, respectively) aiming at euthyroidism [1, 27, 36–38]. Hypothyroidism is the goal for RAIT, also in children, and thus risks will be lower both in persistent/recurrence disease and in developing thyroid neoplasm in non-irradiated thyroid tissue [27, 39–43].

The second goal is to reduce gland volume (in particular in patients with medium gland volume), thereby correcting both mechanical issues (e.g., dysphagia, dyspnea) and anti-esthetic features of the neck [44].

The success of RAIT is mainly linked to both radioiodine administered activity (and its kinetics in the gland: i.e., effective half-life) and thyroid volume, as already demonstrated [1, 27, 45–48].

According to the *"function oriented concept"* an adsorbed dose of 150 Gy is necessary to obtain euthyroidism [27, 49].

On the contrary, obtaining hyperthyroidism correction according to the *"ablative dose concept"* (i.e., hypothyroidism), it is necessary to deliver an absorbed dose ranging from 200 to 300 Gy to the target [27, 37, 49, 50]. The frequency of persistent hyperthyroidism is very low (8%) delivering an adsorbed dose close to 300 Gy to the target [37].

However, Krohn and colleagues [51], in their retrospective analysis, reported how not the total thyroid absorbed dose but the maximum dose rate (≥2.2 Gy/h) may be important to achieve hypothyroidism. To date, however, their preliminary data have to be confirmed by prospective studies.

Finally, in pediatric GD patients, the absorbed dose for delivery to target should range from 120 Gy to 300 Gy [39, 52–54].

Strategies that can be used to choose radioiodine activity, to obtain the adsorbed dose reported above, are described in the specific section.

Since RAI can produce an increase of serum thyroid hormone levels, patients should be treated in a euthyroid state, discontinuing ATD (i.e., MMI, carbimazole or propylthiouracil)

a few days (2–5) before RAIT, thus reducing the risk of the so-called *"thyroid storm."* This approach may be more important in elderly patients and/or in patients with comorbidities (e.g., cardiovascular, cerebrovascular, systemic or pulmonary hypertension, renal failure) [1, 24, 55–59]. ß-Adrenergic block drugs should be used accurately both before and after RAIT [60, 61]. Finally, if possible, the use of ATD should be avoided in the days/weeks after RAIT since they can reduce therapy efficacy, as already demonstrated [24].

2.2.3 Toxic Multinodular Goiter (TMNG) or Toxic Adenoma (TA)

RAIT is a safe, effective therapeutic option for toxic (multi)-nodular goiter patients [29].

TMNG or TA patients may undergo RAIT as first option care if: (1) they have a solitary hyperfunctioning nodule; (2) they have multiple hyperfunctioning nodules in multinodular goiter without suspected or confirmed thyroid cancer; (3) they are advanced in age; (4) they have comorbidities (e.g., cardiovascular, cerebrovascular, systemic or pulmonary hypertension) that produce higher surgery risks; (5) they have a previous history of surgery and/or irradiation of neck; and (6) there is limited or no access to a high volume thyroid surgeon [1].

TMNG or TA patient are not advised to undergo RAIT if: (1) they are pregnant or breastfeeding; (2) they have suspected or confirmed thyroid cancer; (3) they have large TMNG; and (4) there are signs and/or symptoms of compression on neck structures [1].

In TMNG or TA patients, the goal of RAIT is to correct the hyperthyroid status (subclinical or overt), restoring euthyroidism. In addition, as a second goal, it is possible to improve mechanical issues (i.e., dysphagia, dyspnea) reducing the volume of toxic thyroid nodule(s) and/or thyroid goiter (if extranodular thyroid parenchyma is not suppressed) by 35% within three months, and up to 45% over 24 months after RAIT [44, 62, 63]. If RAIT is aimed at the latter objective, the use of rhTSH in both TMNG and nontoxic-MNG patients produces greater thyroid volume reduction. In addition, the use of rhTSH may be useful in TMNG with low RAIU values. However, its use is off-label and in TMNG patients could produce an exacerbation of hyperthyroidism [46, 48, 64–69].

Also in TMNG and TA patients, the success rate of RAIT is mainly linked to both radioiodine administered activity (and its kinetics in toxic thyroid nodule(s): i.e., maximum RAIU uptake and effective half-life) and thyroid volume, as already demonstrated [1, 70].

In particular, higher RAI activities quickly produce resolution of hyperthyroidism (more than 70% of TA patients are no longer hyperthyroid 3 months after RAIT) even if the risk of developing early hypothyroidism is higher [1, 71]. However, the incidence of hypothyroidism increases over time and regards about 60% of treated TA patients in the 20 years following RAIT [71–75]. The risk of hypothyroidism is higher for treated patients >45 years old, with higher RAIU, partial suppression of extra toxic thyroid nodule(s) parenchyma and pre-treated with ATD (since they normalize serum TSH levels) [73]. Similarly, also in TMNG patients, the incidence of hypothyroidism increases over time, regarding about 64% of all patients in the 24 years following RAIT (many of them having undergone two or more RAIT) [74].

On the contrary, the risk of persistent or recurrent hyperthyroidism in TMNG patients is higher than in other patients, reaching up to 20% of all treated patients, as already reported [1, 44, 62, 76, 77].

To correct hyperthyroidism, it is necessary to deliver an absorbed dose to the target(s) that ranges from 150 to 300 Gy [27, 78–81]. Higher absorbed doses (i.e., up to 400 Gy) slightly improved the success rate of RAIT in an already published comparative study [81].

Overall, in these patients, the success rate (i.e., definitive correction of hyperthyroidism) is very high, ranging from 81% to 94% of TMNG and TA patients, respectively [1, 27, 44, 78–81].

Strategies that can be used to choose radioiodine activity, to obtain the adsorbed dose reported above, are described in the specific section.

Since RAI may produce a temporary worsening of hyperthyroidism, ß-adrenergic block drugs should be used both in elderly patients and in patients with comorbidities (even if asymptomatic). For the same reason, and in the same patients' setting, it may be useful to reassume ATD some days (3–7) after RAIT (1).

2.2.4 Strategies to Perform RAIT

As is known, the aim of RAIT is to achieve a non-hyperthyroid status reaching euthyroidism in both TA and TMNG patients, or definitive hypothyroidism in GD patients.

However, choosing the best radioiodine activity to definitively correct hyperthyroidism avoiding hypothyroidism in TA and TMNG patients, avoiding persistent/recurrent hyperthyroidism in GD patients, and, finally, reducing the radiation dose to the body (in particular to stomach and bladder) is a challenge because it is not possible to evaluate all of the variables affecting outcome in both the early and late phases.

There is an ongoing debate regarding the optimal approach to use in clinical practice to choose the radioiodine activity that can be administered: first, the so-called "fixed dose" method, an estimation method usually based on evaluation of either the gland or nodule(s) size by palpation, thyroid ultrasonograhy (TUS) measurement or thyroid scintigraphy (TS); second, the "calculation dose" method, a dosimetric, tailored, approach based on RAIU and gland/nodule(s) volume calculation by TUS rather than TS [27, 49].

In daily practice, both methods have advantages and disadvantages. The more relevant advantages of the "fixed dose" method are linked to its simplicity in terms of pretreatment procedures, for both physicians and patients. Generally, a fixed dose between 370–555 and 370–740 MBq is used to treat patients affected by GD and TA/TMNG, respectively [1, 25]. On the contrary, this method, lacking diagnostic accuracy during pretreatment procedures, runs the risk of under- or, mainly, over-treatment, as already described [82].

Thus, taking literature data into account, the cumulative incidence of persistence/recurrence hyperthyroidism (in particular in GD and TMNG) or, on the contrary, of hypothyroidism (in particular in TA without extranodular parenchyma suppression) may also be due to an inaccuracy of the *"fixed dose"* method [44, 72, 73].

The *"calculated dose"* method is used mainly in young patients (<45 years), with the aim to determine the optimal RAI activity to administer to achieve the highest success rate, reducing, at the same time, the adsorbed dose to both normal thyroid parenchyma (i.e., non-target tissue in TA and TMNG patients) and whole body (in particular to so-called *"critical organs"*, such as stomach and bladder), thus respecting the *"as low as reasonably achievable"* (ALARA) principle and the European Union Council Directive (97/43/EURATOM) [49, 83–85].

The *"calculated dose"* method is based on both a measured volume of the gland (GD patients) or nodule(s) (TA or TMNG patients) by TS (planar and SPET images) or, better, TUS and RAIU [25, 27, 49].

The activity to be administered should be calculated as already reported in the European Nuclear Medicine Association guidelines [27].

Recently, Amato and Campennì [70] proposed calculating both the *"net"* volume of hot nodule(s) by subtracting the volume of involution area(s) always evaluated by TUS (thereby reducing the total amount of treated volume and, consequently, the prescribed activity) and RAIU comprising three uptake assessments (3 to 6–24—168 h) to improve diagnostic accuracy of the *"calculated method."*

The main disadvantage of the *"calculated dose"* method may be its complexity for both physicians and patients. However, a simplified calculated dose approach, at least for the treatment of GD patients, has been proposed by using 99mTc- scintigraphy [86, 87].

In conclusion, to date, there is no agreement on the superiority of the *"calculated dose"* over the *"fixed dose"* method [37, 72, 82, 84, 88–92] in the treatment of hyperthyroid patients.

However, according to the latest evidence in literature, use of the *"calculated dose"* method should be preferred in children to young-adult patients, to increase the success rate and,

mainly, to reduce both the incidence of hypothyroidism or persistent/recurrent disease and unjustified radiation exposure to patients, relatives, and non-family environments [27, 50, 93–97].

Finally, the most recent European Union Council Directive (EUROTOM 13/59) has indicated personalized dosimetry (i.e., the *"calculated dose"* method) as the preferred approach to perform nuclear medicine therapies.

2.3 Adverse Effects of Radioactive Iodine Therapy (RAIT)

Despite RAI therapy being a safe and generally well-tolerated treatment, either acute or late side effects may occur, principally related to insufficient clinical control of hyperthyroidism and active thyroid orbitopathy [98]. Indeed, uncontrolled hyperthyroidism and severe active thyroid orbitopathy can be considered as relative contraindications to RAI treatment [99]. Main side effects are summarized in Table 2.4.

2.3.1 Early Side Effects

Early side effects can occur immediately or during the first week after RAI treatment. They are mainly related to thyroid volume and hyperthyroidism control before RAI treatment.

2.3.1.1 Thyroid Swelling
Patients with large goiter after RAI therapy could manifest thyroid pain and sensation of thyroid growth due to inflammation process caused by irradiation of thyroid tissue. In some cases, even if very rare, in patients with both toxic and nontoxic goiter an acute thyroid enlargement for edema could cause tracheal compression and dyspnea.

For example, the use of Recombinant Human Thyrotropin (rh-TSH) administration to enhance RAI effect in nontoxic goiter was associated with more frequent tracheal compression with stridorous respiration [100].

Table 2.4 Summary of early and late side effects

Side effect	Onset	Pathophysiology	Symptoms	Therapy
Thyroid swelling	Early	Inflammatory reaction to irradiation	Thyroid pain Sensation of thyroid growth Dyspnea in patients with large goiter.	It solves in short time without medical intervention; Treatment with nonsteroidal anti-inflammatory agent for 24–48 h after RAI administration can be indicated Corticosteroids could be beneficial.
Radiation thyroiditis and post-therapy thyrotoxicosis	Early	Transient rise in fT3 and fT4 levels	Exacerbation of hyperthyroidism symptoms. Thyroid storm (rare): – high fever – central nervous system manifestations, gastrointestinal and hepatic manifestations – heart failure.	Good selection of the optimal time point of RAI treatment administration Beta-adrenergic blockade ATDs therapy before or after RAI treatment in patient with uncontrolled hyperthyroidism Thyroid storm requires advanced medical treatment with ATDs, inorganic iodide administration beta-AAs, corticosteroids and antipyretics.
Radioiodine-Induced sialadenitis	Early/late	Concentration in salivary of iodide due to the sodium iodine symporter expression	Swelling, Periductal pressure Duct constriction Pain Xerostomia Taste dysfunctions	Lemon juice (5 mL) or salivation-inducing snacks (lemon candy) Start 24 h following RAI therapy
Immunogenic effects	Early	Release of thyroid antigens from destroyed follicular cells with increase of TRAb,	RAI therapy causes the transient increase of TRAb.	Pretreatment with ATDs
Hypothyroidism: transient or persistent	Late	Transient hypothyroidism: unclear cause Persistent hypothyroidism: Thyroid irradiation	Transient hypothyroidism: no symptoms or sign, only biochemical. Persistent hypothyroidism: Typical sign of hypothyroidism	Transient hypothyroidism spontaneously recovers in few months Persistent hypothyroidism requires administration of Levo-thyroxine replacement therapy.
Graves' orbitopathy	Late	B-cells and macrophages activation with cytokines secretion	Worsening or appearance of orbitopathy	In case of **high risk to develop/worsening** of orbitopathy: prophylactic steroids oral administration: daily dose (daily 0.3–0.5 mg prednisone/kg for 15–30 days starting after RAI treatment) In case of **mild** GO: local treatment such as artificial tears and also a 6 months selenium supplementation is supplementation are suggested. In case of **moderate to severe** active GO: intravenous administration steroids is suggested – intermediate-dose protocol with methylprednisolone: – starting dose of 0.5 g once weekly for 6 weeks, followed by 0.25 g once weekly for 6 weeks, – high-dose protocol with methylprednisolone:starting dose of 0.75 g once weekly for 6 weeks followed by 0.5 g once weekly for 6 weeks), both with a cumulative dose that should not exceed 8.0 g. Contraindications: recent viral hepatitis, psychiatric disorders, advanced cardiovascular disease and hepatic dysfunction, diabetes and hypertension. Second-line treatment: rehabilitative surgery.

Table 2.4 (continued)

Side effect	Onset	Pathophysiology	Symptoms	Therapy
Cancer incidence	Late	Irradiation of thyroid tissue, bone marrow, bladder	No significant data are available on cancer incidence after RAI therapy for benign conditions.	There is no evidence of increased risk of RAI induced malignancy Tailored dosimetry and patient education can limit the risk
Teratogenicity and gonadic function	Late	Irradiation of gonadic cells	No increased risk of long-term infertility, miscarriage, induced abortions, stillbirths, or offspring neonatal mortality or congenital defects. Transient reduction of testosterone and T/LH ratio.	Pregnancy represents an absolute contraindication to RAI therapy Testing on blood sample for pregnancy is recommended before RAI treatment Conception should be delayed: in women for 4–6 months or longer in men at least for 3–4 months

To avoid this rare side effect in patients with large volume goiter, surgery is still the first therapeutic option if feasible.

The lack of controlled trial and the great inter-individual variations do not allow a prophylactic therapy strategy in large goiter, but in case of moderate thyroid swelling or tenderness, these symptoms usually vanish in short time without medical intervention. Nevertheless, in some cases treatment with nonsteroidal anti-inflammatory agent for 24–48 hours after RAI administration can be indicated to limit symptoms and the use of corticosteroids could also be probably beneficial.

2.3.1.2 Radiation Thyroiditis and Post-therapy Thyrotoxicosis

Radiation thyroiditis may occur in 1% of patients during the first weeks after RAI and it could be associated with a transient rise in free Triiodothyronine (fT3) and free Tiroxine (fT4) levels that, in patients with poorly controlled hyperthyroidism before RAI, could lead to exacerbation of symptoms up to the so-called "thyroid storm" [29].

Thyroid storm is rare but it is a life-threatening condition regarding decompensations of multiple organs with high fever, central nervous system manifestations, gastrointestinal and hepatic manifestations, and heart failure [56, 101]. It requires comprehensive and advanced medical treatment with the administration of antithyroid drugs (ATDs), inorganic iodide, beta-adrenergic

receptor antagonists (beta-AAs) corticosteroids, and antipyretics [101].

If thyroid storm is a rare condition, in the early period after RAI a mild to severe worsening of thyrotoxicosis occurs in 10% of patients [58]. In particular, patients with poorly controlled hyperthyroidism are most likely at risk to present this condition. A good selection of the optimal time point of RAI treatment administration and a correct premedication are mandatory to limit these side effects.

A beta-adrenergic blockade if not already installed and in the absence of contraindication has to be implemented after RAI treatment to avoid cardiac side effect such as tachycardia or cardiac arrhythmia.

The antithyroid drugs (ATDs) are frequently used in the treatment management of this condition to accelerate the return to an euthyroidism status but there is disagreement about the effects of their administration before or after RAI therapy. Pretreatment with ATD allows these patients to start from a lower baseline value of thyroid hormones, but RAI efficacy can be compromised and a most rapid increase in thyroid hormone levels can be observed [58].

Pretreatment with ATDs, in particular Carbimazole, could decrease iodine uptake with a higher risk of treatment failure, despite underlying mechanism is not fully understood. In particular, it reduces the cell damage produced by synthesis of oxygen free radicals subsequent to RAI administration [102]. A withdrawal of

Carbimazole for only a few days before RAI administration is enough both to restore the success of RAI and to avoid the risk of exacerbation of hyperthyroidism.

Also pretreatment with propylthiouracil (PTU) is associated with an higher risk of RAI therapy failure [103]. In a study conducted in 1997 [103] this risk of treatment failure was statistically significant after discontinuation of PTU for 4–7 days before RAI ($P = 0.039$), while it was not significant after discontinuation for longer than a week. Others authors [104] suggested that PTU administration should be avoided in patients with Graves' disease before RAI administration because it could lead to higher risk of treatment failure compared to methimazole (MMI) administration or absence of any therapy ($P < 0.05$). A systematic review published in 2007 compared the rates of treatment failure and the short- and long-term side effects in patients with hyperthyroidism treated with RAI with or without adjunctive ATDs and found out that the risk of treatment failure defined as persistent or recurrent hyperthyroidism or need for further RAI treatment was significantly higher in adjunctive ATDs group compared with control ($P = 0.006$); no significant differences were found between different ATDs [24].

Several studies investigated the potential role of lithium administration. The concomitant administration of lithium with RAI could lead to a better control of hyperthyroidism [105], probably related to the lithium-induced blockade of RAI and thyroid hormone release, without effect on thyroidal RAI uptake [106, 107], and it may also prevent worsening of thyrotoxicosis after ATDs interruption or RAI therapy [108], but it is not routinely used.

To avoid the decrease of RAI efficacy in case of persistent thyreotoxicosis it is suggested to reintroduce soon ATDs after RAI administration [24].

Radiation thyroiditis like subacute thyroiditis should be treated also with nonsteroidal anti-inflammatory agents as anti-inflammatory action: corticosteroids should be used when patients fail to respond to nonsteroidal anti-inflammatory drugs or present initially with moderate to severe pain and/or thyrotoxic symptoms [1].

Sometimes it is difficult to differentiate between post-therapy thyrotoxicosis and persistent hyperthyroidism for treatment failure: RAI reaches the goal in 3–6 months and delayed response to treatment can be confused as persistent/transient thyrotoxicosis. No-responders patients to RAI treatment usually continue to manifest the same symptoms and signs of thyrotoxicosis, so in cases of persistent hyperthyroidism 3 months after RAI patients could be retreated with a second dose of RAI [109].

2.3.1.3 Radioiodine-Induced Sialadenitis

Sialadenitis represents both an acute and a late side effect of RAI therapy and it is one of the most frequent complication in case of RAI treatment for thyroid cancer ablation, while it is less frequent after RAI treatment for Graves' disease or toxic goiter.

Salivary gland can concentrate iodide due to the sodium iodine symporter expression and then secrete into saliva [110]. This mechanism is principally mediated by ductal epithelium of parotid gland and during this process salivary glands are exposed to dose-related damage.

Clinical manifestations of radioiodine-induced sialadenitis, transient in more cases, are swelling and pain, xerostomia or taste dysfunctions, mainly represented by salty taste for reduction of reabsorption of sodium and chloride from the saliva, [110] in as many as 20–30% of cases [111].

Swelling increases periductal pressure with duct constriction and obstructive symptoms for the formation of jelly-like plug [110] secondary to obstruction and mucus precipitation that often increases in the eating period.

Because this common side effect can affect quality of life of patients, several authors proposed various radioprotective procedures to diminish RAI damage to salivary gland.

A valid method is the stimulation by lemon juice that lead to a faster secretion from salivary gland [112]: after administration of 5 mL of lemon juice, RAI in salivary gland declined in 4 min, followed by a re-accumulation period of 20–40 min of the same initial activity.

Another method is the assumption of salivation-inducing snacks, like lemon candy [113], starting 24 h following RAI therapy. On the other hand an early administration of lemon juice or substitutes is not recommended because of increased side effects on salivary gland function [114] because acid stimulation increases not only salivary flow, but also salivary gland blood flow and RAI uptake in iodine-avid tissue rises up in 24 h and then reaches a plateau [113]. Subsequent continuous assumption of lemon juice or similar helps RAI clearance from the salivary glands.

2.3.1.4 Immunogenic Effects

Various therapeutic approaches such ATDs, RAI, or thyroidectomy for hyperthyroidism condition may influence disease activity. Normally during follow-up, TSH receptor antibodies (TRAb) level tend to disappear from serum after all types of therapeutic modalities [115].

On the other hand, radioactive iodine therapy could induce a transient increase of TRAb secondary to the release of thyroid antigens from destroyed follicular cells and this event is more evident during the first days after RAI administration. Patients that underwent surgery or ATDs showed a gradual fall of TRAb in serum and after 1 year 50–60% of patients demonstrated the disappearance of TRAb. Underlying mechanism of TRAb reduction in not well established: one hypothesis is that hyperthyroid state may maintain autoimmune abnormalities while euthyroid state after medication or surgery decrease autoimmune reaction with decrease in TRAb levels [115].

No correlation has been found between the entity of TRAb rise neither with RAI activity administered nor with baseline fT3 and fT4 levels [116]. TRAb levels rise occurred as a generalized phenomenon, despite corticosteroids prophylaxis after RAI.

The incidence of immunogenic hyperthyroidism/Graves' disease after RAI therapy for autonomous nodules has been described [117] and this risk has also been associated to high levels of thyroid peroxidase (TPO) antibodies before RAI administration [118], fitting the hypothesis that

immunogenic hyperthyroidism in these patients represents an exacerbation of a preexisting and occult immunogenic thyroid disorder.

An aggravating factor of thyroid immunity in addition to autoantibodies expression is the reduction of T-lymphocyte suppressor after RAI simultaneously to a rise of both pro-inflammatory and anti-inflammatory cytokines [98].

The most serious consequence of re-activation of thyroid immunity after RAI therapy with severe impact to patient's quality life is the activation or new onset of Graves' orbitopathy (GO) [98]. A period of pretreatment with ATDs may diminish the TRAb rise after RAI [119, 120] contributing to the suppression of TSH receptor antibodies with their immunosuppressive action. Furthermore methimazole probably interferes with antigen macrophages processing, leading to decreased T cell response and antibodies production [120].

2.3.2 Late Side Effects

2.3.2.1 Hypothyroidism: Transient or Persistent

The great part of patients can develop hypothyroidism after RAI treatment, especially after high-doses administration, and it could be both transient and persistent. Even if it is counted among side effects, hypothyroidism in most cases is considered the goal of the treatment.

Transient hypothyroidism may manifest 2–5 months after RAI therapy and spontaneously recover in few months without development of symptoms or sings of hypothyroidism: a predominant problem is to differentiate from permanent type in early months after treatment to establish the best treatment option. The cause remains unclear and no prognostic factors have been identified to predict its onset [121].

Authors suggest different hypothesis in pathogenesis of transient hypothyroidism.

Several authors speculated that thyroid-stimulating antibody (TSAb) may play a role in recovery of follicular cells function after RAI [121, 122], so the measurement of TSAb levels could early differentiate transient hypothyroidism to permanent one. Thyroid-stimulating antibody levels could decrease after several months and patients could develop permanent hypothyroidism, furthermore the mean estimated time to develop permanent hypothyroidism is shorter compared to patients with transient hypothyroidism: for these reasons a strict follow-up is needed in these patients.

Other authors [123] supposed that an impaired thyroid function could be secondary to hibernation-like conditions (or stunning). Patients with transient hypothyroidism may manifest an impaired organification of iodide, with normal iodide trapping by the thyroid; on the other hand, in patients with permanent hypothyroidism, iodide trapping is markedly diminished and do not recover. To discriminate transient versus permanent hypothyroidism, early iodine uptake measurements may be useful to establish substitutive therapy.

Finally, other authors suggested that transient hypothyroidism is caused by an hypothalamic-pituitary axis dysfunction [124], like recovery delay, but subsequent studies did not confirm this hypothesis [125].

2.3.2.2 Graves' Orbitopathy

Graves' orbitopathy (GO) is an inflammatory autoimmune disorder linked to thyroid disease due to several antigens shared between orbital and thyroid tissue [126] as T-lymphocytes. T-lymphocytes reach orbital tissue and interact with antigens exposed by B-cells and macrophages activating several reactions like cytokines secretion that maintain orbital fibroblasts proliferation and extraocular infiltration muscles with increased volume of orbital content [11, 127].

Furthermore, orbital fibroblasts express TSH receptors that represent the primary target for TRAb, working like autoantigen and worsening inflammatory reactions [128].

TRAb are expressed by the most part of patients with Graves' disease, including euthyroid ones. Generally, high TRAb levels are associated with a more aggressive orbitopathy and worse prognosis [129–131].

Several studies demonstrated a significant association between RAI therapy and worsening or development of ophthalmopathy. A recent systematic review [132] compared its occurrence in patients treated with thyroidectomy, ATDs, or RAI. This review included nine studies with a total of 1773 patients and found out that RAI therapy represents a significant risk to develop/worse orbitopathy compared to ATDs ($P < 0.00001$). Prophylactic per os or by intravenous administration of steroids has been demonstrated effective in preventing this event ($P = 0.002$), especially in patients with prior orbitopathy.

Several concomitant risk factors, beyond high TRAb levels, are associated with the development or deterioration of orbitopathy, such as smoking, high fT3 levels, and post-RAI hypothyroidism [133, 134].

In particular, cigarette smoking has been investigated by several authors as a major independent risk factor involved in ophthalmopathy. A systematic review [135] including 15 studies with a total of 1880 patients underlined the strong association between smoking and orbitopathy, despite biological mechanism remaining unknown. Moreover, smoking had been demonstrated to be associated with poor outcome even in case of prophylactic administration of steroids after RAI therapy, but also in case of radiation therapy and high-dose i.v. glucocorticoid treatment in patients with severe ophthalmopathy [133]. For these reasons smoking cessation should be encouraged in all patients with Graves' disease, especially with orbitopathy.

Thyroid function is also a crucial point to consider for development or deterioration of orbitopathy. Both hypothyroidism and hyperthyroidism conditions must be avoided: in fact hypothyroidism after RAI therapy for Graves' disease represent a risk factor for ophthalmopathy; for this reason early (after 2 weeks from RAI) substitutive therapy with levothyroxine has been proposed to prevent this event [134]. On the other hand, also high pretreatment fT3 levels must be avoided: serum concentration ≥ 5 nmol per liter has associated with development or worsening of orbitopathy [136].

Selection of the best therapy option is based on activity and severity of GO. Activity is measured by the clinical activity score (CAS) [137] that considered seven clinical criteria: spontaneous retrobulbar pain, pain on attempted upward or downward gaze, redness of eyelids, redness of conjunctiva, swelling of caruncle or plica, swelling of eyelids, and chemosis. Active GO is defined when CAS point is major or equal to 3/7.

Severity is classified as mild, moderate to severe, and sight threatening (or very severe). Mild GO is defined when orbitopathy have a minor impact on daily life and does not requires therapy, moderate-to-severe GO is defined when orbitopathy requires immunosuppression or surgical treatment and very severe GO that requires immediate intervention, is defined when patients present dysthyroid optic neuropathy (DON) and/or corneal breakdown [138].

In 2016 the European Group on Graves' Orbitopathy (EUGOGO) published the guidelines for the management of GO [139]. They recommended that patients with GO should be referred to specialized centers with both endocrinologist and ophthalmological expertises, to stop smoking attitude should be recommended even in absence of GO and euthyroid status should be promptly restored and maintained in patients with severe GO, RAI treatment should not be the first therapeutic option. If other treatment option are not feasible, in patients at high risk of development/worsening of orbitopathy and candidate to RAI treatment prophylactic steroids oral administration are recommended, starting with a daily dose of 0.3–0.5 mg prednisone/kg after body weight per day. Original schedule suggested to continue steroid prophylaxis for 3 months after treatment [139, 140], but subsequently was shown that a lower daily dose of 0.2 mg prednisone/kg body weight per day for 6 weeks was equally effective [139].

On the other hand, in low-risk patients lower doses can be used while patients with inactive orbitopathy may receive RAI without steroid cover.

For mild GO local treatment, artificial tears and a 6 months selenium supplementation that has demonstrated improvement in eye manifestation are suggested. A large multicenter, double-blind study published in 2011 [141] demonstrated that a supplementation with sodium selenite (100 μg twice daily, corresponding to 93.6 μg of elemental selenium/day) significantly improved not only quality of life and overall ocular involvement in the selenium group, but also the rate of progression of GO to more severe forms was significantly lower in selenium group versus placebo group ($P < 0,001$).

Guidelines by EUGOGO group [139] recommended intravenous administration of steroids only in moderate to severe active GO with the exception of patients with recent viral hepatitis, psychiatric disorders, advanced cardiovascular disease and hepatic dysfunction and with particular regard to patients with diabetes and hypertension. They proposed both intermediate-dose and high-dose protocols of methylprednisolone, with a starting dose of 0.5 g once weekly for 6 weeks, followed by 0.25 g once weekly for 6 weeks and a starting dose of 0.75 g once weekly for 6 weeks, followed by 0.5 g once weekly for 6 weeks, respectively, both with a cumulative dose that should not exceed 8.0 g. Patients should be monitored to evaluate response to treatment and to early identify possible adverse events of steroids to considerer other treatment modality.

Second-line treatment for moderate to severe and active GO include rehabilitative surgery (for example orbital decompression) when orbitopathy is associated with visual disfunction, and in case of dysthyroid optic neuropathy (DON) onset, it must be suddenly treated with very high dose of steroids (500 mg–1 g of methylprednisolone) for three consecutive days or on alternate days during the first week and proceed with orbital decompression in case of no or poor response after 2 weeks of high-dose steroids protocol.

2.3.2.3 Cancer Incidence

Few data are available on cancer incidence after RAI therapy for benign conditions in adults. Data available on higher activities employed for treatment in patients with thyroid cancer are not reliable, due to different RAI pharmacodynamics and pharmacokinetics related to the absence of thyroid gland in these patients [98].

A study published in 2007 [142] evaluated the cancer incidence in 2793 patients with hyperthyroidism treated with RAI, with an average follow-up of 10 years and reported a higher risk of cancer development in patients treated with RAI compared to control population (rate ratio [RR], 1.25). Moreover an increased incidence of kidney (RR, 2.32), stomach (RR, 1.75), and breast (RR, 1.53) cancer was reported in RAI group with relative risk of cancer increasing with higher RAI doses.

A subsequent study suggested that hyperthyroidism itself is a serious clinical condition that could lead to an increased incidence of mortality, independently from treatment modality [143]. Furthermore, although the data suggested a small increase in the risk of upper gastrointestinal cancer in elderly men, other risk factors particularly relevant in these tumors were not recorded, such as smoking history, dietary history, or family history. In this study data about increased risk of leukemia or thyroid cancer after RAI treatment are also not available [143]. On the other hand, one issue is the risk of thyroid cancer after exposure to RAI in childhood.

It is known that the thyroid gland of children, is especially sensitive to the carcinogenic action of ionizing radiation, with a direct relationship between dose of radiation and effect, especially for lower dose levels (on the order of 0.10 Gy), compared to higher dose levels that resulted in cell killing [1, 144]. Carcinogenic effect of RAI exposure of children remains uncertain.

A paper published in 2005 [145] analyzed the risk of thyroid cancer in 276 patients younger than 15 years at the time of Chernobyl nuclear power plant accident in April 1986 and investigated other concomitant factors that could possibly influence this risk. A direct relationship between radiation dose to the thyroid and thyroid cancer risk was found ($P < 0.001$); moreover the risk of radiation-related thyroid cancer was three times higher in iodine-deficient areas (relative risk [RR] = 3.2, 95% CI = 1.9–5.5) than elsewhere indicating that use of a dietary iodine supplement can reduce the risk of RAI-related thyroid cancer.

In 2007 a study was performed to identify both risk and benefits of RAI treatment, compared with other therapies for hyperthyroidism condition due to Graves' disease in children [42]: this study concluded that, if properly adminis-

tered, RAI remains an ideal treatment modality for Graves' disease in the pediatric population and that higher rather than lower doses of RAI should be given for the increased risk of thyroid cancer associated with low dose of RAI, as previously described.

Another study [146] with a long follow-up (36 years) analyzed 116 patients, aged of 3–19 years, treated with RAI for Graves' disease between 1953 and 1973. Despite the small sample size resulting in an inadequate statistical power, no thyroid cancer or leukemia and no increase in the rate of spontaneous abortion or in the number of congenital anomalies were reported.

In 2007 a conflicting study [147] suggested to perform surgery instead of RAI both in children and in young adults for lacking of long-term, prospective, randomized control trials. Other reasons to support surgery instead of RAI are the potential risk of internal and external radiation exposures inducing hyperparathyroidism and the slightly higher cardiovascular and overall mortality rates induced by RAI compared to patients not receiving RAI.

Furthermore [148], thyroid cancer risk may be associated with the underlying thyroid disease and a tailored dosimetry and patient education are necessary.

Nevertheless at this moment RAI treatment is still considered a valid option to treat hyperthyroidism in children because there is no a clear evidence of increased risk of RAI-induced malignancy. International guidelines do not recommend RAI Treatment only in very young children (<5 years).

2.3.2.4 Teratogenicity and Gonadic Function

Radiation is known to be mutagenic and the majority of studies focused on pregnancy outcome and gonadic function after RAI regards only patients treated for thyroid carcinoma.

Pregnancy represents an absolute contraindication to RAI therapy and a pregnancy test on blood sample is recommended 72 h before RAI administration [1, 27].

Fetal thyroid begins to develop at 5–6 weeks and colloid production begins at 10–12 weeks of gestation: inadvertent RAI therapy administration before 10 weeks of gestation has been associated with normal fetus [149]; on the other hand, a later administration results in high thyroid radiation dose (20–600 Gy) with thyroid ablation and neonatal hypothyroidism [98].The rate of induced abortion, miscarriage, stillbirth, prematurity, birth weight below the tenth percentile for the gestational age, congenital abnormality, and death during the first year of life was investigated in 2008 in a study on 2673 pregnancies in patients treated with RAI for thyroid cancer without significant external radiation to the ovaries [150]. Incidence of miscarriages was 10% before any treatment for thyroid cancer and frequency was not significantly higher in women treated with RAI during the year before conception, even in case of higher activity administration. Also the incidence of stillbirths, prematurity, low birth weight, congenital malformations, and death during the first year of life were not significantly different before and after RAI therapy, and incidences of thyroid and non-thyroid cancers were similar in children born either before or after the mother's exposure to radioiodine.

A systematic review published in 2008 [151] evaluated the gonadic and reproductive effects of RAI therapy in women and adolescents survivor from thyroid cancer between 8 and 50 years treated with RAI at various activities ranging from 1110 to 40,663 MBq. Transient amenorrhea occurred in 8–27% of women within the first year after RAI, particularly in older women. In addition, patients treated with RAI experienced menopause at a slightly younger age than women not treated with RAI.

Also this review confirmed that RAI treatment for thyroid cancer was generally not associated with a significantly increased risk of long-term infertility, miscarriage, induced abortions, stillbirths, or offspring neonatal mortality or congenital defects. This result can be translated in a certain safety of RAI treatment for hyperthyroidism.

Radiation dose absorbed by the testis after a single ablative dose of RAI is lower than to the ovaries and it is below that associated with permanent damage to germinal epithelium, so the risk of infertility in these patients is minimal, also in patients that underwent multiple administrations for persistent or metastatic thyroid cancer [152].

The effects of RAI treatment for hyperthyroidism on male gonadal function was investigated in one study [153]. Nineteen male hyperthyroid patients were enrolled, seventeen with Graves' disease and two with toxic adenoma, and demonstrated a significant reduction of both serum testosterone (T) ($P = 0.04$) and T/LH ratio ($P = 0.007$) 45 days after RAI with return to basal levels after 12 months. A significant increase in progressive motility after RAI therapy was observed ($P = 0.01$) without significant variations in sperm concentration and percentage of normal forms. In conclusion RAI treatment for hyperthyroidism has a minor impact on gonadic function and it should keep in mind that also thyroid dysfunctions may affected sperm quality and motility [154]. Based on recommendation for RAI treatment in thyroid cancer, also in case of RAI treatment for hyperthyroidism it would be better to delay conception in women for 4–6 months or longer until euthyroidism is reached and in men at least for 3–4 months to allow turnover of sperm production [143].

References

1. Ross DS, Burch HB, Cooper DS, Greenlee MC, Laurberg P, Maia AL, et al. 2016 American thyroid association guidelines for diagnosis and management of hyperthyroidism and other causes of thyrotoxicosis. Thyroid. 2016;26(10):1343–421.
2. Biondi B, Cooper DS. The clinical significance of subclinical thyroid dysfunction. Endocr Rev. 2008;29:76–131.
3. Burch HB. Overview of the clinical manifestations of thyrotoxicosis. In: Werner SC, Ingbar SC, editors. The thyroid. Philadelphia: Lippincott Williams & Wilkins; 2013. p. 434–40.
4. Cooper DS. Hyperthyroidism. Lancet. 2003; 362(9382):459–68.
5. Flynn RW, Macdonald TM, Morris AD, et al. The thyroid epidemiology, audit, and research study: thyroid dysfunction in the general population. J Clin Endocrinol Metab. 2004;8989:3879–84.
6. Nyström HF, Jansson S, Berg G. Incidence rate and clinical features of hyperthyroidism in a long-term iodine sufficient area of Sweden (Gothenburg) 2003–2005. Clin Endocrinol. 2013;78(5):768–76.

7. Laurberg P, Bulow PI, Knudsen N, et al. Environmental iodine intake affects the type of non-malignant thyroid disease. Thyroid. 2001;11:457–69.

8. Smith TJ, Hegedüs L. Graves' disease. N Engl J Med. 2016;375:1552–65.

9. Bartalena L, Masiello E, Magri F, Veronesi G, Bianconi E, Zerbini F, et al. The phenotype of newly diagnosed Graves' disease in Italy in recent years is milder than in the past: results of a large observational longitudinal study. J Endocrinol Investig. 2016;39:1445–51.

10. Ruggeri R, Giuffrida G, Campennì A. Autoimmune endocrine disease. Minerva Endocrinol. 2018; 43(3):305–22.

11. Bahn RS. Mechanisms of disease: Graves' ophthalmopathy. N Engl J Med. 2010;362(2):726–38.

12. Cooper G, Bynum M, Somers E. Recent insights in the epidemiology of autoimmune diseases: improved prevalence estimates and understanding of clustering of diseases. J Autoimmun. 2009;33:197–207.

13. Boelaert K, Newby P, Simmonds M, Holder R, Carr-Smith J, Heward J, et al. Prevalence and relative risk of other autoimmune diseases in subjects with autoimmune thyroid disease. Am J Med. 2010;123:183. e1–9.

14. Ruggeri R, Trimarchi F, Giuffrida G, Certo R, Cama E, Campennì A, et al. Autoimmune comorbidities in Hashimoto's thyroiditis: different patterns of association in adulthood and childhood/adolescence. Eur J Endocrinol. 2017;176(2):133–41.

15. Aghini-Lombardi F, Antonangeli L, Martino E, et al. The spectrum of thyroid disorders in an iodinedeficient community: the Pescopagano survey. J Clin Endocrinol Metab. 1999;84:561–6.

16. Ruggeri R, Campennì A, Sindoni A, Baldari S, Trimarchi F. Benvenga. Association of autonomously functioning thyroid nodules with Hashimoto's thyroiditis: study on a large series of patients. Exp Clin Endocrinol Diabetes. 2011;119(10):621–7.

17. Giovanella L, D'Aurizio F, Campenni A, Ruggeri R, Baldari S, Verburg F, et al. Searching for the most effective thyrotropin (TSH) threshold to rule-out autonomously functioning thyroid nodules in iodine deficient regions. Endocrine. 2016;54:757–61.

18. Gozu H, Lublinghoff J, Bircan R, Paschke R. Genetics and phenomics of inherited and sporadic nonautoimmune hyperthyroidism. Mol Cell Endocrinol. 2010;322:125–34.

19. Tonacchera M, Chiovato L, Pinchera A, Agretti P, Fiore E, Cetani F, et al. Hyperfunctioning thyroid nodules in toxic multinodular goiter share activating thyrotropin receptor mutations with solitary toxic adenoma. J Clin Endocrinol Metab. 1998;83(2):492–8.

20. Vicchio T, Giovinazzo S, Certo R, Cucinotta M, Micali C, Baldari S, et al. Lack of association between autonomously functioning thyroid nodules and germline polymorphisms of the thyrotropin receptor and gas genes in a mild to moderate iodine-deficient caucasian population. J Endocrinol Investig. 2017;37:625–30.

21. Boelaert K, Torlinska B, Holder R, Franklyn J. Older subjects with hyperthyroidism present with a paucity of symptoms and signs: a large cross-sectional study. J Clin Endocrinol Metab. 2010;95(6):2715–26.

22. Frost L, Vestergaard P, Mosekilde L. Hyperthyroidism and risk of atrial fibrillation or flutter: a population-based study. Arch Intern Med. 2004;164(15):1675–8.

23. Ruggeri R, Trimarchi F, Biondi B. MANAGEMENT OF ENDOCRINE DISEASE: l-Thyroxine replacement therapy in the frail elderly: a challenge in clinical practice. Eur J Endocrinol. 2017; 177(4):R199–217.

24. Walter MA, Briel M, Christ-Crain M, Bonnema SJ, Connell J, Cooper DS, et al. Effects of antithyroid drugs on radioiodine treatment: systematic review and meta-analysis of randomised controlled trials. BMJ. 2007;334(7592):514.

25. Jolanta MD, Bogsrud TV. Nuclear medicine in evaluation and therapy of nodular thyroid. In: Thyroid nodules. Switzerland: Springer International; 2018.

26. Silberstein E, Alavi A, Balon H, Clarke S, Divgi C, Gelfand MJ, et al. The SNMMI practice guideline for therapy of thyroid disease with 131I 3.0. J Nucl Med. 2012;53(10):1633–51.

27. Stokkel MPM, Handkiewicz Junak D, Lassmann M, Dietlein M, Luster M. EANM procedure guidelines for therapy of benign thyroid disease. Eur J Nucl Med Mol Imaging. 2010;37(11):2218–28.

28. Brzozowska M, Roach P. Timing and potential role of diagnostic I-123 scintigraphy in assessing radioiodine breast uptake before ablation in postpartum women with thyroid cancer: a case series. Clin Nucl Med. 2006;31(11):683–7.

29. Ross DS. Radioiodine therapy for hyperthyroidism. N Engl J Med. 2011;364:543–50.

30. Bartalena L, Chiovato L, Vitti P. Management of hyperthyroidism due to Graves' disease: frequently asked questions and answers (if any). J Endocrinol Investig. 2016;39(10):1105–14.

31. Bahn R, Burch H, Cooper D, Garber J, Greenlee M, Klein I, et al. Hyperthyroidism and other causes of thyrotoxicosis: management guidelines of the American thyroid association and american association of clinical endocrinologists. Thyroid. 2011;21(6):593–646.

32. Träisk F, Tallstedt L, Abraham-Nordling M, Andersson T, Berg G, Calissendorff J, et al. Thyroid-associated ophthalmopathy after treatment for Graves' hyperthyroidism with antithyroid drugs or iodine-131. J Clin Endocrinol Metab. 2009;94(10):3700–7.

33. Eckstein AK, Plicht M, Lax H, Neuhäuser M, Mann K, Lederbogen S, et al. Thyrotropin receptor autoantibodies are independent risk factors for graves' ophthalmopathy and help to predict severity and outcome of the disease. J Clin Endocrinol Metab. 2006;91(9):3464–70.

34. Reiners C. Radioactivity and thyroid cancer. Hormones. 2009;8:185–92.

35. Ron E, Doody M, Becker D, Harris B 3rd, Hoffman D, McConahey WM, et al. Cancer mortality following treatment for adult hyperthyroidism. Cooperative thyrotoxicosis therapy follow- up study group. JAMA. 1998;280:347–55.

36. Kobe C, Eschner W, Sudbrock F, Weber I, Marx K, Dietlein M, et al. Graves' disease and radioiodine therapy: is success of ablation dependent on the achieved dose above 200 Gy? Nuklearmedizin. 2008;47:13–7.

37. Reinhardt MJ, Brink I, Joe A, Von Mallek D, Ezziddin S, Palmedo H, et al. Radioiodine therapy in Graves' disease based on tissue-absorbed dose calculations: effect of pre-treatment thyroid volume on clinical outcome. Eur J Nucl Med. 2002;29:1118–24.

38. Dunkelmann S, Neumann V, Staub U, Groth P, Kuenstner H, Schuemichen C. Results of a risk adapted and functional radioiodine therapy in Graves' disease. Nuklearmedizin. 2005;44:238–42.

39. Rivkees S. Controversies in the management of Graves' disease in children. J Endocrinol Investig. 2016;39(11):1247–57.

40. Dobyns B, Sheline G, Workman J, Tompkins E, McConahey W, Becker D. Malignant and benign neo- plasms of the thyroid in patients treated for hyperthyroidism: a report of the cooperative thyrotoxicosis therapy follow-up study. J Clin Endocrinol Metab. 1974;38:976–98.

41. Sheline GE, McCormack K, Galante M. Thyroid nodules occurring late after treatment of thryotoxicosis with radioiodine. J Clin Endocrinol Metab. 1962;22:8–17.

42. Rivkees SA, Dinauer C. An optimal treatment for pediatric Graves' disease is radioiodine. J Clin Endocrinol Metab. 2007;92(3):797–800.

43. Chao M, Jiawei X, Guoming W, Jianbin L, Wanxia L, Driedger A, et al. Radioiodine treatment for pediatric hyperthyroid Graves' disease. Eur J Pediatr. 2009;168:1165–9.

44. Tarantini B, Ciuoli C, Di Cairano G, Guarino E, Mazzucato P, Montanaro A, et al. Effectiveness of radioiodine (131-I) as definitive therapy in patients with autoimmune and non-autoimmune hyperthyroidism. J Endocrinol Investig. 2006;29(7):594–8.

45. Kung A, Yau C, Cheng A. The action of methimazole and L-thyroxine in radioiodine therapy: a prospective study on the incidence of hypothyroidism. Thyroid. 1995;5:7–12.

46. Bonnema SJ, Bennedbæk FN, Veje A, Marving J, Hegedüs L. Propylthiouracil before 131I therapy of hyperthyroid diseases: effect on cure rate evaluated by a randomized clinical trial. J Clin Endocrinol Metab. 2004;89(9):4439–44.

47. Santos R, Romaldini J, Ward L. A randomized controlled trial to evaluate the effectiveness of 2 regimens of fixed iodine (131I) doses for Graves disease treatment. Clin Nucl Med. 2012;37:241–4.

48. Braga M, Walpert N, Burch H, Solomon B, Cooper D. The effect of methimazole on cure rates after radioiodine treatment for Graves' hyperthyroidism: a randomized clinical trial. Thyroid. 2002;12:135–9.

49. Hänscheid H, Canzi C, Eschner W, Flux G, Luster M, Strigari M, et al. 2013 EANM Dosimetry committee series on standard operational procedures for pre-therapeutic dosimetry II. Dosimetry prior to radioiodine therapy of benign thyroid diseases. Eur J Nucl Med Mol Imaging. 2013;40:1126–34.

50. Willegaignon J, Sapienza M, Buchpiguel CA. Radioiodine therapy for Graves disease: thyroid absorbed dose of 300 Gy-tuning the target for therapy planning. Clin Nucl Med. 2013;38(4):231–6.

51. Krohn T, Hänscheid H, Müller B, Behrendt F, Heinzel A, Mottaghy F, et al. Maximum dose rate is a determinant of hypothyroidism after 131i therapy of Graves' disease but the total thyroid absorbed dose is not. J Clin Endocrinol Metab. 2014;99(11):4109–15.

52. Rivkees SA, Sklar C, Freemark M. Clinical review 99: the management of Graves' disease in children, with special emphasis on radioiodine treatment. J Clin Endocrinol Metab. 1998;83(11):3767–76.

53. Goolden A, Davey J. The ablation of normal thyroid tissue with iodine-131. Br J Radiol. 1963;36:340–5.

54. Graham G, Burman K. Radioiodine treatment of Graves' disease. An assessment of its potential risks. Ann Intern Med. 1986;105:900–5.

55. McDermott M, Kidd G, Dodson LJ, Hofeldt F. Radioiodine-induced thyroid storm. Case report and literature review. Am J Med. 1983;75:353–9.

56. Akamizu T, Satoh T, Isozaki O, Suzuki A, Wakino S, Iburi T, et al. Diagnostic criteria, clinical features, and incidence of thyroid storm based on nationwide surveys. Thyroid. 2012;22(7):661–79.

57. Shafe R, Nuttall F. Acute changes in thyroid function in patients treated with radioactive iodine. Lancet. 1975;2:635–7.

58. Burch HB, Solomon BL, Cooper DS, Ferguson P, Walpert N, Howard R. The effect of antithyroid drug pretreatment on acute changes in thyroid hormone levels after 131I ablation for Graves' disease. J Clin Endocrinol Metab. 2001;86(7):3016–21.

59. Andrade V, Gross J, Maia A. Effect of methimazole pretreatment on serum thyroid hormone levels after radioactive treatment in Graves' hyperthyroidism. J Clin Endocrinol Metab. 1999;84:4012–6.

60. Klein I, Danzi S. Thyroid disease and the heart. Circulation. 2007;116:1725–35.

61. Klein I. Endocrine disorders and cardiovascular disease. In: Libby P, et al., editors. Braunwald's heart disease: a textbook of cardiovascular medicine. 8th ed. Philadelphia: Saunders/Elsevier; 2008. p. 2033–47.

62. Nygaard B, Hegedus L, Ulriksen P, Nielsen K, Hansen J. Radioiodine therapy for multinodular toxic goiter. Arch Intern Med. 1999;159:1364–8.

63. Bonnema S, Bertelsen H, Mortensen J, Andersen P, Knudsen D, Bastholt L, et al. The feasibility of high

dose iodine 131 treatment as an alternative to surgery in patients with a very large goiter: effect on thyroid function and size and pulmonary function. J Clin Endocrinol Metab. 1999;84:3636–41.

64. Lee Y, Tam K, Lin Y, Leu W, Chang J, Hsiao C, et al. Recombinant human thyrotropin before (131) I therapy in patients with nodular goitre: a meta-analysis of randomized controlled trials. Clin Endocrinol. 2015;83:702–10.

65. Nieuwlaat W, Hermus A, Sivro-Prndelj F, Corstens F, Huysmans D. Pretreatment with recombinant human TSH changes the regional distribution of radioiodine on thyroid scintigrams of nodular goiters. J Clin Endocrinol Metab. 2001;86:5330–6.

66. Silva M, Rubió I, Romão R, Gebrin E, Buchpiguel C, Tomimori E, et al. Administration of a single dose of recombinant human thyrotrophin enhances the efficacy of radioiodine treatment of large compressive multinodular goitres. Clin Endocrinol. 2004;60:300–8.

67. Nielsen V, Bonnema S, Hegedus L. Transient goiter enlargement after administration of 0.3 mg of recombinant human thyrotropin in patients with benign non-toxic nodular goiter: a randomized, double- blind, cross-over trial. J Clin Endocrinol Metab. 2006;91:1317–22.

68. Nielsen V, Bonnema S, Boel-Jorgensen H, Grupe P, Hegedus L. Stimulation with 0.3 mg recombinant human thyrotropin prior to iodine 131 therapy to improve the size reduction of benign non-toxic nodular goiter: a prospective randomized double-blind trial. Arch Intern Med. 2006;166:1476–82.

69. Nieuwlaat W, Huysmans D, Van den Bosch HC, Sweep CG, Ross H, Corstens F, et al. Pretreatment with a single, low dose of recombinant human thyrotropin allows dose reduction of radioiodine therapy in patients with nodular goiter. J Clin Endocrinol Metab. 2003;88:3121–9. J Clin Endocrinol Metab. 2003;88:3121–9.

70. Amato E, Campennì A, Leotta S, Ruggeri R, Baldari S. Treatment of hyperthyroidism with radioiodine targeted activity: a comparison between two dosimetric methods. Phys Med. 2016;32(6):847–53.

71. Zakavi S, Mousavi Z, Davachi B. Comparison of four different protocols of I-131 therapy for treating single toxic thyroid nodule. Nucl Med Commun. 2009;30:169–75.

72. Metso S, Jaatinen P, Huhtala H, Luukkaala T, Oksala H, Salmi J. Long-term follow-up study of radioiodine treatment of hyperthyroidism. Clin Endocrinol. 2004;61:641–8.

73. Ceccarelli C, Bencivelli W, Vitti P, Grasso L, Pinchera A. Outcome of radioiodine-131 therapy in hyperfunctioning thyroid nodules: a 20 years' retrospective study. Clin Endocrinol. 2005;62:331–5.

74. Holm L, Lundell G, Israelsson A, Dahlqvist I. Incidence of hypothyroidism occurring long after iodine-131 therapy for hyperthyroidism. J Nucl Med. 1982;23:103–7.

75. Yano Y, Sugino K, Akaishi J, Uruno T, Okuwa K, Shibuya H, et al. Treatment of autonomously functioning thyroid nodules at a single institution: radioiodine therapy, surgery, and ethanol injection therapy. Ann Nucl Med. 2011;25:749–54.

76. Erickson D, Gharib H, Li H, Van Heerden J. Treatment of patients with toxic multinodular goiter. Thyroid. 1998;8:277–82.

77. Kang A, Grant C, Thompson G, Van Heerden J. Current treatment of nodular goiter with hyperthyroidism (Plummer's disease): surgery versus radioiodine. Surgery. 2002;132:916–23.

78. Reinhardt M, Joe A, Von Mallek D, Zimmerlin M, Manka-Waluch A, Palmedo H, et al. Dose selection for radioiodine therapy of borderline hyperthyroid patients with multifocal and disseminated autonomy on the basis of 99mTc-pertechnetate thyroid uptake. Eur J Nucl Med Mol Imaging. 2002;29:480–5.

79. Dunkelmann S, Endlicher D, Prillwitz A, Rudolph F, Groth P, Schuemichen C. Results of a TcTUs-optimized radioiodine therapy of multifocal and disseminated functional thyroid autonomy. Nuklearmedizin. 1999;38:131–9.

80. Reiners C, Schneider P. Radioiodine therapy of thyroid autonomy. Eur J Nucl Med. 2002;29(Suppl 2):S471–8.

81. Reinhardt M, Kim B, Wissmeyer M, Juengling F, Brockmann H, Von Mallek D, et al. Dose selection for radioiodine therapy of borderline hyperthyroid patients according to thyroid uptake of 99mTc-pertechnetate: applicability to unifocal thyroid autonomy? Eur J Nucl Med Mol Imaging. 2006;33:608–12.

82. Allahabadia A, Daykin J, Sheppard M, Gouch S, Franklyn J. Radioiodine treatment of hyperthyroidism—prognostic factors for outcome. J Clin Endocrinol Metab. 2001;86(8):3611–7.

83. ICRP (1987). Protection of the patient in nuclear medicine (and statement from the 1987 Como Meeting of ICRP). ICRP Publication 52. Ann. ICRP 17 (4). ICRP Publ 52 Ann ICRP 17 (4). 1987;

84. Sisson J, Anca M, Avram A, Rubello D, Milton D, Gross M. Radioiodine treatment of hyperthyroidism: fixed or calculated doses; intelligent design or science? Eur J Nucl Med Mol Imaging. 2007;34:1129–30.

85. European Union Council Directive 97/43/EURATOM on health protection of individuals against the dangers of ionising radiation in relation to medical exposure. Luxembourg: Council of the European Union. 1997. http://ec.europa.eu/energy/nuclear/radioprotection/doc/legislation/9743_en.pdf.

86. Szumowski P, Mojsak M, Abdelrazek S, Sykala M, Filonowicz A, Dorota Jurgilewicz D, et al. Calculation of therapeutic activity of radioiodine in Graves' disease by means of Marinelli's formula, using technetium (99mTc) scintigraphy. Endocrine. 2016;54:751–6.

87. Giovanella L, Verburg F, Ceriani L. One-stop-shop radioiodine dosimetry in patients with Graves' disease. Endocrine. 2017;56(1):220–1.

88. De Rooij A, Vandenbroucke J, Smit J, Stokkel M, Dekkers O. Clinical outcomes after estimated versus calculated activity of radioiodine for the treatment of hyperthyroidism: systematic review and meta-analysis. Eur J Endocrinol. 2009;161(5):771–7.

89. Leslie W, Ward L, Salamon E, Ludwig S, Rowe R, Cowden E. A randomized comparison of radioiodine doses in Graves' hyperthyroidism. J Clin Endocrinol Metab. 2003;88:978–83.

90. Peters H, Fischer C, Bogner U, Reiners C, Schleusener H. Treatment of Graves' hyperthyroidism with radioioidine; results of a prospective study. Thyroid. 1997;2:247–51.

91. Alexander EK, Larsen PR. High dose ^{131}I therapy for the treatment of hyperthyroidism caused by Graves' disease. J Clin Endocrinol Metab [Internet]. 2002;87(3):1073–7. https://doi.org/10.1210/jcem.87.3.8333.

92. Kendall-Taylor P, Keir M, Ross W. Ablative radioiodine therapy for hyperthyroidism: long term follow up study. Br Med J. 1984;289:361–3.

93. Vija Racaru L, Fontan C, Bauriaud-Mallet M, Brillouet S, Caselles O, Zerdoud S, et al. Clinical outcomes 1 year after empiric 131I therapy for hyperthyroid disorders: real life experience and predictive factors of functional response. Nucl Med Commun. 2017;38(9):756–63.

94. Liu B, Tian R, Peng W, He Y, Huang R, Kuang A. Radiation safety precautions in 131I therapy of Graves' disease based on actual biokinetic measurements. J Clin Endocrinol Metab. 2015;100(8):2934–41.

95. Rokni H, Sadeghi R, Moossavi Z, Treglia G, Zakavi S. Efficacy of different protocols of radioiodine therapy for treatment of toxic nodular goiter: systematic review and meta-analysis of the literature. Int J Endocrinol Metab. 2014;12(2):e14424.

96. Willegaignon J, Sapienza M, Coura-Filho G, Watanabe T, Traino A, Buchpiguel C. Graves' disease radioiodine-therapy: choosing target absorbed doses for therapy planning. Med Phys. 2014;41(1):12503.

97. Cooper J. International commission on radiological protection. 2012 radiation protection principles. J Radiol Prot. 2012;32(1):N81–7.

98. Bonnema SJ, Hegedüs L. Radioiodine therapy in benign thyroid diseases: effects, side effects, and factors affecting therapeutic outcome. Endocr Rev. 2012;33(6):920–80.

99. De Leo S, Lee SY, Braverman LE. Hyperthyroidism. Lancet. 2016;388(10047):906–18.

100. Bonnema SJ, Nielsen VE, Boel-Jørgensen H, Grupe P, Andersen PB, Bastholt L, et al. Improvement of goiter volume reduction after 0.3 mg recombinant human thyrotropin-stimulated radioiodine therapy in patients with a very large goiter: a double-blinded, randomized trial. J Clin Endocrinol Metab. 2007;92(9):3424–8.

101. Satoh T, Isozaki O, Suzuki A, Wakino S, Iburi T, Tsuboi K, et al. 2016 Guidelines for the management of thyroid storm from The Japan Thyroid Association and Japan Endocrine Society (First edition). Endocr J. 2016;63(12):1025–64.

102. Walter MA, Christ-Crain M, Schindler C, Müller-Brand J, Müller B. Outcome of radioiodine therapy without, on or 3 days off carbimazole: a prospective interventional three-group comparison. Eur J Nucl Med Mol Imaging. 2006;33(6):730–7.

103. Hancock LD, Tuttle RM, LeMar H, Bauman J, Patience T. The effect of propylthiouracil on subsequent radioactive iodine therapy in Graves' disease. Clin Endocrinol. 1997;47(4):425–30.

104. Santos RB, Romaldini JH, Ward LS. Propylthiouracil reduces the effectiveness of radioiodine treatment in hyperthyroid patients with Graves' disease. Thyroid. 2004;14(7):525–30.

105. Bogazzi F, Bartalena L, Brogioni S, Scarcello G, Burelli A, Campomori A, Manetti L, Rossi G, Pinchera AME. Comparison of radioiodine with radioiodine plus lithium in the treatment of Graves' hyperthyroidism. J Clin Endocrinol Metab. 1999;84:499–503.

106. Robbins J. Perturbations of iodine metabolism by lithium. Math Biosci. 1984;72:337–47.

107. Temple R, Berman M, Robbins JWJ. The use of lithium in the treatment of thyrotoxicosis. J Clin Invest. 1972;51:2746–56.

108. Bogazzi F, Bartalena L, Campomori A, Brogioni S, Traino C, De Martino F, et al. Treatment with lithium prevents serum thyroid hormone increase after thionamide withdrawal and radioiodine therapy in patients with graves' disease. J Clin Endocrinol Metab. 2002;87(10):4490–5.

109. Gayed I, Wendt J, Haynie T, Dhekne R, Moore W. Timing for repeated treatment of hyperthyroid disease with radioactive iodine after initial treatment failure. Clin Nucl Med. 2001;26(1):1–5.

110. Mandel SJ, Mandel L. Radioactive iodine and the salivary glands. Thyroid. 2003;13(3):265–71.

111. Grewal RK, Larson SM, Pentlow CE, Pentlow KS, Gonen M, Qualey R, et al. Salivary gland side effects commonly develop several weeks after initial radioactive iodine ablation. J Nucl Med. 2009;50(10):1605–10.

112. Van Nostrand D, Bandaru V, Chennupati S, Wexler J, Kulkarni K, Atkins F, et al. Radiopharmacokinetics of radioiodine in the parotid glands after the administration of lemon juice. Thyroid. 2010;20(10):1113–9.

113. Nakada K, Ishibashi T, Takei T, Hirata K, Shinohara K, Katoh S, et al. Does lemon candy decrease salivary gland damage after radioiodine therapy for thyroid cancer? J Nucl Med. 2005;46(2):261–6.

114. Jentzen W, Balschuweit D, Schmitz J, Freudenberg L, Eising E, Hilbel T, et al. The influence of saliva flow stimulation on the absorbed radiation dose to the salivary glands during radioiodine therapy of thyroid cancer using 124I PET(/CT) imaging. Eur J Nucl Med Mol Imaging. 2010;37(12):2298–306.

115. Laurberg P, Wallin G, Tallstedt L, Abraham-Nordling M, Lundell G, Törring O. TSH-receptor autoimmunity in Graves' disease after therapy with anti-thyroid drugs, surgery, or radioiodine: a 5-year prospective randomized study. Eur J Endocrinol. 2008;158(1):69–75.

116. Chiappori A, Villalta D, Bossert I, Ceresola EM, Lanaro D, Schiavo M, et al. Thyrotropin receptor autoantibody measurement following radiometabolic treatment of hyperthyroidism: comparison between different methods. J Endocrinol Investig. 2010;33(3):197–201.

117. Schmidt M, Gorbauch E, Dietlein M, Faust M, Stützer H, Eschner W, et al. Incidence of postradioiodine immunogenic hyperthyroidism/Graves' disease in relation to a temporary increase in thyrotropin receptor antibodies after radioiodine therapy for autonomous thyroid disease. Thyroid. 2006;16(3):281–8.

118. Nygaard B, Knudsen JH, Hegedüs L, Veje AH. Thyrotropin receptor antibodies and Graves' disease, a side effect of 131I treatment in patients with nontoxic goiter. J Clin Endocrinol Metab. 1997;82:2926–30.

119. Gamstedt A, Wadman B, Karisson A. Methimazole, but not betamethasone, prevents 131 I treatment-induced rises in thyrotropin receptor autoantibodies in hyperthyroid Graves' disease. J Clin Endocrinol Metab. 1986;62:773–7.

120. Andrade VA, Gross JL, Maia AL. Serum thyrotropin-receptor autoantibodies levels after I therapy in Graves' patients: effect of pretreatment with methimazole evaluated by a prospective, randomized study. Eur J Endocrinol. 2004;151:467–74.

121. Aizawa Y, Yoshida K, Kaise N, Fukazawa H, Kiso Y, Sayama N, et al. The development of transient hypothyroidism after iodine-131 treatment in hyperthyroid patients with Graves' disease: prevalence, mechanism and prognosis. Clin Endocrinol. 1997;46(1):1–5.

122. Sawers JSA, Toft AD, Irvine WJ, Brown NS, Seth J. Transient hypothyroidism after iodine-131 treatment of thyrotoxicosis. J Clin Endocrinol Metab. 1980;50:226–9.

123. Connell JM, Hilditch TE, McCruden DCAW. Transient hypothyroidism following radio-iodine therapy for thyrotoxicosis. Br J Radiol. 1983;56(665):309–13.

124. Uy HL, Reasner CA, Samuels MH. Pattern of recovery of the hypothalamic-pituitary-thyroid axis following radioactive iodine therapy in patients with Graves' disease. Am J Med. 1995;99(2):173–9.

125. Gómez N, Gómez JM, Orti A, Gavaldà L, Villabona C, Leyes P, Soler J. Transient hypothyroidism after iodine-131 therapy for Grave's disease. J Nucl Med. 1995;36(9):1539–42.

126. Bartalena L, Fatourechi V. Extrathyroidal manifestations of Graves' disease: a 2014 update. J Endocrinol Investig. 2014;37(8):691–700.

127. Smith T. Pathogenesis of Graves' orbitopathy: a 2010 update. J Endocrinol Investig. 2010;33:414–21.

128. Iyer S, Bahn R. Immunopathogenesis of Graves' ophthalmopathy: the role of the TSH receptor. Best Pract Res Clin Endocrinol Metab. 2012;26(3):281–9.

129. Bahn RS, Dutton CM, Joba W, Heufelder AE. Thyrotropin receptor expression in cultured Graves' orbital preadipocyte fibroblasts is stimulated by thyrotropin. Thyroid. 1998;8:193–6.

130. Lytton SD, Ponto KA, Kanitz M, Matheis N, Kohn LD, Kahaly GJ. A novel thyroid stimulating immunoglobulin bioassay is a functional indicator of activity and severity of Graves' orbitopathy. J Clin Endocrinol Metab. 2010;95:2123–31.

131. Gerding MN, van der Meer JW, Broenink M, Bakker O, Wiersinga WM, Prummel MF. Association of thyrotrophin receptor antibodies with the clinical features of Graves' ophthalmopathy. Clin Endocrinol. 2000;52:267–71.

132. Li HX, Xiang N, Hu WK, Jiao XL. Relation between therapy options for Graves' disease and the course of Graves' ophthalmopathy: a systematic review and meta-analysis. J Endocrinol Investig. 2016;39(11):1225–33.

133. Bartalena L, Marcocci C, Tanda ML, Manetti L, Dell'Unto E, Bartolomei MP, et al. Cigarette smoking and treatment outcomes in Graves ophthalmopathy. Ann Intern Med. 1998;129(8):632–5.

134. Stan MN, Bahn RS. Risk factors for development or deterioration of Graves' ophthalmopathy. Thyroid. 2010;20(7):777–83.

135. Thornton J, Kelly SP, Harrison RA, Edwards R. Cigarette smoking and thyroid eye disease: a systematic review. Eye. 2007;21(9):1135–45.

136. Tallstedt L, Lundell G, Tørring O, Wallin G, Ljunggren JG, Blomgren H, Taube A. Occurrence of ophthalmopathy after treatment for Graves' hyperthyroidism. N Engl J Med. 1992;326:1733–8.

137. Mourits M, Prummel M, Wiersinga W, Koornneef L. Clinical activity score as a guide in the management of patients with Graves´ ophthalmopathy. Clin Endocrinol. 1997;47(1):9–14.

138. Bartalena L, Baldeschi L, Dickinson AJ, Eckstein A, Kendall-Taylor P, Marcocci C, et al. Consensus statement of the European group on Graves' orbitopathy (EUGOGO) on management of Graves' orbitopathy. Thyroid. 2008;18(3):333–46.

139. Bartalena L, Baldeschi L, Boboridis K, Eckstein A, Kahaly GJ, Marcocci C, et al. The 2016 European Thyroid Association/European Group on Graves' orbitopathy guidelines for the management of graves' orbitopathy. Eur Thyroid J. 2016;5(1):9–26.

140. Bartalena L, Marcocci C, Bogazzi F, Manetti L, Tanda M, Dell'Unto E, et al. Relation between therapy for hyperthyroidism and the course. N Engl J Med. 1998;338:73–8.

141. Marcocci C, Kahaly GJ, Krassas GE, Bartalena L, Prummel M, Stahl M, Altea MA, Nardi M, Pitz S, Boboridis K, Sivelli P, von Arx G, Mou-rits MP, Baldeschi L, Bencivelli W, Wiersinga W, European Group on Graves' Orbitopathy. Selenium and the

course of mild Graves' orbitopathy. N Engl J Med. 2011;364:1920–31.

142. Metso S, Auvinen A, Huhtala H, Salmi J, Oksala H, Jaatinen P. Increased cancer incidence after radioiodine treatment for hyperthyroidism. Cancer. 2007;109(10):1972–9.

143. Vanderpump M. Cardiovascular and cancer mortality after radioiodine treatment of hyperthyroidism. J Clin Endocrinol Metab. 2007;92(6):2033–5.

144. Boice JD. Radiation-induced thyroid cancer - What's new? J Natl Cancer Inst. 2005;97(10):703–5.

145. Cardis E, Kesminiene A, Ivanov V, Malakhova I, Shibata Y, Khrouch V, et al. Risk of thyroid cancer after exposure to 131I in childhood. J Natl Cancer Inst. 2005;97(10):724–32.

146. Read CH Jr, Tansey MJ, Menda Y. A 36-year retrospective analysis of the efficacy and safety of radioactive iodine in treating young Graves' patients. J Clin Endocrinol Metab. 2004;89:4229–33.

147. Lee JA, Grumbach MM, Clark OH. The optimal treatment for pediatric Graves' disease is surgery. J Clin Endocrinol Metab. 2007;92(3):801–3.

148. Lucignani G. Long-term risks in hyperthyroid patients treated with radioiodine: is there anything new? Eur J Nucl Med Mol Imaging. 2007;34(9):1504–9.

149. Berg G, Jacobsson L, Nyström E, Gleisner KS, Tennvall J. Consequences of inadvertent radioiodine treatment of Graves' disease and thyroid cancer in undiagnosed pregnancy. Can we rely on routine pregnancy testing? Acta Oncol. 2008;47(1):145–9.

150. Garsi J-P, Schlumberger M, Rubino C, Ricard M, Labbe M, Ceccarelli C, et al. Therapeutic administration of 131I for differentiated thyroid cancer: radiation dose to ovaries and outcome of pregnancies. J Nucl Med. 2008;49(5):845–52.

151. Sawka AM, Lakra DC, Lea J, Alshehri B, Tsang RW, Brierley JD, et al. A systematic review examining the effects of therapeutic radioactive iodine on ovarian function and future pregnancy in female thyroid cancer survivors. Clin Endocrinol. 2008;69(3):479–90.

152. Hyer S, Vini L, O'Connell M, Pratt B, Harmer C. Testicular dose and fertility in men following L131 therapy for thyroid cancer. Clin Endocrinol. 2002;56(6):755–8.

153. Ceccarelli C, Canale D, Battisti P, Caglieresi C, Moschini C, Fiore E, et al. Testicular function after 131I therapy for hyperthyroidism. Clin Endocrinol. 2006;65(4):446–52.

154. Krassas GE, Pontikides N. Male reproductive function in relation with thyroid alterations. Best Pract Res Clin Endocrinol Metab. 2004;18(2):183–95.

Radioiodine Therapy of Thyroid Cancer

3

Frederik A. Verburg

3.1 Introduction

3.1.1 Differentiated Thyroid Cancer

Although it concerns fewer than 1% of all cancer cases, and its incidence varies throughout the world [1], differentiated thyroid carcinoma (DTC) is the most common endocrine malignancy [2]. This comprises the so-called papillary thyroid carcinoma (PTC) and follicular thyroid carcinoma (FTC). These tumours derive from the follicular thyrocytes and are referred to as "differentiated" thyroid cancer because the tumour cells retain some of normal thyrocytes' properties. Most importantly the ability to take up and store iodine and to respond to thyrotropin (thyroid-stimulating hormone, TSH) stimulation is retained, which allows for treatment and imaging using radioactive iodine analogues. DTC cases typically have a good prognosis, with long-term survival ranging from about 70% to more than 95%, depending on the extent of disease at the time of diagnosis [3]. Consequently, in >85% of DTC patients, life expectancy is unimpaired [4, 5].

3.1.1.1 Histology and Clinical Behaviour

PTC

The classical form of PTC is an unencapsulated tumour with papillary and follicular structures. It is characterized by overlapping cell nuclei that have a ground-glass appearance and longitudinal grooves, with invaginations of cytoplasm into the nuclei [6, 7]. PTC histologic variants among others include the encapsulated, follicular, tall-cell, columnar cell, clear-cell, diffuse sclerosing, solid or trabecular, and oxyphilic forms [2, 8]. PTCs are often multifocal, with many of the lesions of different clonal origin, i.e. arising independently [9]. PTC metastasis tends to be lymphogenic, before spreading to the lungs and bones.

FTC

FTC is characterized by follicular differentiation, without the nuclear changes seen in PTC [6, 7]. FTCs are encapsulated tumours, distinguishable from follicular adenomas by the presence of invasion of the capsule and/or vessels. According to the pattern of invasion, FTCs can be divided into two categories: minimally invasive and widely invasive. FTCs are less often multifocal than are PTCs. FTC tends to metastasize to the lungs, bone and liver; regional lymph node metastases are much less common than in PTC.

Hürthle cell carcinoma is a variety of FTC that consists of at least 75% oxyphilic cells [8]. An important characteristic of Hürthle cell carcinomas

F. A. Verburg (✉)
Department of Nuclear Medicine, University Hospital Marburg, Marburg, Germany
e-mail: verburg@med.uni-marburg.de

is their reputedly poor or even absent iodine uptake, which renders this entity more difficult to treat.

3.1.1.2 DTC Treatment

In the treatment of DTC, multiple modalities are involved, each of which will be discussed separately.

Surgery

Surgery is the first and most important component of the primary treatment of DTC. In Europe, the Americas, and much of Australasia, (near) total thyroidectomy is usually performed in almost all patients. Only for papillary microcarcinoma hemithyroidectomy is deemed to suffice by most patients [9–17].

The most serious potential complications of thyroid surgery are hypoparathyroidism and recurrent laryngeal nerve damage [18, 19]. Identification and electronic monitoring of the recurrent laryngeal nerve can significantly reduce the rate of nerve damage [20]. The incidence and impact of complications can be reduced by performing the procedure in expert centres [19] as well as intensive post-operative monitoring, especially serum calcium levels should be monitored frequently in the immediate post-operative phase.

Thyroid Hormone Replacement Therapy

As by definition the production of endogenous thyroxine is discontinued by thyroidectomy procedure, DTC patients require thyroid hormone (levothyroxine, LT4) replacement therapy [21].

Differentiated thyroid cancer cells still react to TSH stimulation; for this reason LT4 in more advanced cases is usually administered in such doses that TSH levels fall to very low levels of <0.1 mU/L [22]. Especially for low-risk patients TSH suppression is not generally advocated [21].

Radioiodine (I-131) Therapy

A landmark study by Mazzaferri and Jhiang published in 1994 on a population of over 1500 patients followed for four decades or more clearly showed that both recurrence rates and death rates related to DTC were much lower in patients who received radioiodine treatment (RIT) after surgery than in those who did not receive I-131 [13]. In fact, now that I-131 therapy belongs to the standard treatment of DTC, life expectancy in patients without extensive neck or distant metastases is unimpaired [4].

I-131-NaI closely approaches the ideal oncologic drug. It is one of the earliest and longest used examples of selective targeted therapy [23]. It can be used both for imaging the drug distribution and for diagnostics and treatment. I-131-NaI is a very specific radiopharmaceutical for targeting cancer cells that have retained the normal thyrocytes' functional attributes as the body's main iodine reservoir and primary locus of expression of the sodium-iodide symporter (NIS) [24], making I-131 largely specific for the target cancer cell.

In clinical practice, post-operative, adjuvant I-131 therapy is primarily applied to destroy remaining occult small DTC foci, thus decreasing the long-term risk of recurrent disease [10, 13, 25–27]. Furthermore, by eliminating remaining normal thyroid tissue the specificity of serum thyroglobulin and diagnostic whole-body scans (dxWBS) as markers for persistent or recurrent DTC are improved [2, 26, 28]. Additionally, given the multiclonal nature of many DTC cases [9] by destroying healthy thyroid cells ablation may prevent neoplastic transformation from occurring again [29]. As an added bonus I-131 ablation allows sensitive post-ablation whole body scanning (rxWBS) for detecting previously unknown persistent locoregional disease or distant metastases [30, 31]. The latter does not however in itself constitute a goal or justification for I-131 ablation.

The effectiveness of I-131 ablation in the prevention of recurrent disease and DTC-related death has been shown sufficiently in multiple studies, especially in high-risk patients or in cases of non-radical surgery [13, 32, 33].

I-131 therapy has been used for treating DTC for over 75 years [23]. However, there still is no agreement on the activity of I-131 to use for which clinical situation, let alone on what parameters to use to determine the activity. As a reflection of this lack of evidence and procedural guidance physicians often still administer standard Iodine-131 dosages as fractions or multiples of "millicuries" although SI-units for the amount of radioactivity have been converted to "Becquerels" more than 30 years ago. Most often I-131 ablation or therapy is administered in the form of a standard activity. The simplest approach to individualize I-131 ablation using fixed activities is the empirical variation of this fixed activity according to stage and histological findings of the surgical specimen. Current guidelines are largely in consensus that the primary goal of initial I-131 therapy, adjuvant post-surgical thyroid remnant ablation, adjuvant treatment or therapy of remaining local or metastatic disease, should influence the therapeutic activity; to what extent is however subject of discussion [34–36]. In children, if no dosimetry is performed, the activity should furthermore be individualized according to body weight, in which the calculation is usually based on an activity per kg bodyweight given to a 70 kg adult [37–39].

3.2 rhTSH

High thyrotropin levels (above 30 mU/L) are usually recommended for I-131 therapy in order to induce sufficient I-131 uptake [34–36]. Such high TSH levels can be achieved either by thyroid hormone withdrawal (THW) for 3–4 weeks or by intramuscular injections of recombinant human TSH. Through avoidance of hypothyroidism, the use of rhTSH results in an unimpaired quality of life [40–42]. A further advantage of rhTSH is that it results in a lower radiation exposure to the remainder of the body, including the bone marrow [43], the reproductive system and the salivary glands [44, 45], thus at least in theory reducing the risk of complications. Over time, many studies have shown the equivalence of rhTSH to THW both for TSH-stimulated Tg testing with or without concurrent dxWBS [46] and for initial I-131 ablation of patients without distant metastases. Furthermore, rhTSH is likely cost-effective from several points of view [47, 48].

3.3 Salivary and Lacrimal Gland Damage (Sicca Syndrome)

One of the most frequent long-term complications of I-131 therapy concerns the salivary glands. As these physiologically take up I-131 as well, in some patients this causes a sufficient irradiation of the organ to cause permanent salivary gland dysfunction. This results in a permanent xerostomia (dry mouth) which severely impairs patients' quality of life.

Attempts have been made to protect the salivary glands during I-131 therapy by the intravenous administration of 500 mg/m^2 S-2-(3-aminopropylamino)-ethylphosphorothioic acid (amifostine) prior to therapy. In a double-blind trial the administration of amifostine leads to an unchanged salivary gland function compared to the pre-therapeutic situation, whereas patients who did not receive amifostine showed a highly significant reduction of the salivary gland function [49]. Treatment with a lower dose of 300 mg/m^2 in a later trial was shown not to be effective [50]. The concept of amifostine protection has not been explored further since, possibly due to potential side effects of the substance.

Traditionally it was thought that stimulation of the salivary glands using, e.g. lemon drops and/or chewing gum would lead to a lower radiation exposure to the salivary glands through an increased washout of I-131 in the excreted saliva. However, several recent studies have shown that this strategy, at least when applied immediately after I-131 administration, may on the contrary lead to an increased radiation exposure through an increase in blood flow to the salivary glands, resulting in an increased I-131 uptake [51]. There is some clinical evidence that delaying the start of stimulation to at least 24 h after the ingestion of I-131 may in fact lead to a lower rate of salivary gland dysfunction [52].

Less known than the damage to the salivary glands is the damage that may be caused to the lacrimal glands by I-131 therapy, the latter occurring with a much lower frequency. Nonetheless, the occurrence of both these phenomena is clearly less frequent subjectively than objectively, with objective xerostomia occurring objectively in the great majority of patients even after only 3.7 GBq I-131 (38/46 patients; [53]) and in all patients after 14.8 GBq or more. However, only a minority of patients complained of this in the lower activity groups. Xerophthalmia was present in a lower percentage of patients (9/46 objectively, 7/46 subjectively after 3.7 GBq I-131 to 3/5 subjectively and 4/5 objectively in patients receiving 14.8 GBq I-131 or more; [53]).

3.4   Malignant Sequellae

Originally hailed in the popular press as a form of magic, it quite soon became evident that even this very specific, targeted drug is not without its long-term side effects and complications. First reports of acute myeloid leukaemia in DTC patients treated with I-131 were already published in the 1950s [54] by the group who first introduced I-131 for DTC. In the ensuing decades, many more scientific publications which examined the role of I-131 in inducing secondary malignancies emerged with differing results: some reports allege that I-131 does induce not only haematological but also possibly solid malignancies [55], whereas others could show that excess non-thyroid malignancy rates are observed in similar heights before as well as after I-131, making a causal relationship with I-131 unlikely [56].

Nonetheless, that exposure to radioactive iodine might cause an increase in the rate of secondary haematological (or other) malignancies is not implausible. I-131 will, after oral or i.v. application, first circulate systemically before being taken up in DTC cells. Well-perfused organs such as the bone marrow are therefore exposed to similar radiation absorbed doses as the blood itself—as was already shown in the 1960s [57]. As the red bone marrow is a highly proliferative tissue, it is also highly sensitive to any DNA-damaging agents or interventions (this is not just limited to radiation, but may also include cytotoxic chemotherapy), which may cause a short-term depression in complete blood cell counts (CBCs) [58, 59]. Furthermore, at least in theory, DNA damage to this highly pro-

liferative tissue may in the long term contribute to the induction of malignant neoplasms.

Recently, new data were published which showed again that it is not unlikely that I-131 therapy of DTC may cause secondary haematological malignancies [60, 61]. Although these reports show a significant increase in the risk of such secondary malignancies, these studies can nonetheless also be regarded as evidence *in support of* radioiodine therapy in DTC. As was detailed in calculations by Piccardo et al. [62], the data presented by Molenaar et al. allow the calculation of the absolute excess risk of haematological malignancies in DTC patients treated with I-131. This risk approximately amounts to one case per ten million patient years [62]. Even assuming that all these cases will result in a fatality—which is hardly likely the case—I-131 may still compare favourably to not giving I-131, e.g. by missing the diagnosis of and thereby timely treatment of distant metastases when this treatment modality is omitted. In fact, this excess risk is so small as likely to be unnoticed in the individual physicians' life-long practice. So small in fact, that it may be less risky in terms of risk of mortality to perform I-131 than to make a patient drive to the attending physicians' office more often, than taking an aspirin [63], or many other environmental risks from daily life.

3.5   Haematological Complications

As detailed above, I-131 may affect the red bone marrow. Not only does this contribute to an elevated risk of secondary haematological malignancies but also to a risk of impairment of bone marrow function. Molinaro et al. detailed in 2009 that one year after I-131 ablation, white blood cell and platelet count was still significantly lower than at baseline, even though the difference was minor and not clinically relevant [58]. Long-term data were not reported by these authors. Verburg et al. reported on the effects of dosimetrically determined high activities of I-131 on blood cell counts and found that, although there was a marked but non-critical effect in the short term, there was no remaining drop in blood cell counts in the long term [59].

3.6 Fertility

Just like the red bone marrow, especially male gonadal tissue cells are highly proliferative and therefore generally susceptible to radiation. From external radiation therapy, it is known that this effect is cumulative.

In men, after I-131 therapy effects like an increased follicle stimulating hormone (FSH), an increased luteinizing hormone (LH) and oligospermia have been described in 20 to >50% of patients receiving high cumulative I-131 activities (13 GBq I-131 and more) [64]. Furthermore, after a single course of I-131 therapy, FSH and LH levels after 6 months are significantly elevated compared to baseline before returning to normal at 18 months post therapy, as an expression of transient impairment of testicular function [64]. Therefore, especially in patients with more advanced disease in whom higher cumulative I-131 activities can be foreseen, pre-therapeutic banking of sperm should be counselled to patients who have or may in the future develop the wish to conceive a child.

With regard to female fertility after I-131 therapy of thyroid cancer, Sawka et al. performed a meta-analysis of 16 studies on this topic [65]. Significant effects described in some studies were the presence of transitory menstrual irregularities, transitory hormonal changes in terms of elevated FSH and LH levels and the earlier, by approximately 1 year, onset of menopause.

3.7 Pulmonary Fibrosis

In patients with extensive lung metastases, and this especially concerns paediatric patients who may show a miliary pulmonary spread at diagnosis, the dose delivered to the lung parenchyma during I-131 therapy of DTC metastases may lead to pulmonary fibrosis, which is a potentially deadly complication of I-131 therapy in paediatric DTC [66]. In order to prevent this, it is advisable to regularly monitor pulmonary function in patients with pulmonary metastases and to refrain from further I-131 therapy in patients in whom a reduction in pulmonary function is suspected. Furthermore, safety of I-131 therapy can be increased by performing a dosimetry before administration of therapy, setting the limit at 3 GBq or 40 MBq per kg body weight whole body retention 48 h after administration of therapy.

References

1. Parkin DM, Muir CS, Whelan SL, Gao YT, Ferlay J, Powell J. In: IARC scientific publications, editor. Cancer incidence in five continents, vol. vol. 6. Lyon, France: International Agency for Research on Cancer; 1992.
2. Schlumberger MJ. Papillary and follicular thyroid carcinoma. N Engl J Med. 1998;338:297–306.
3. Verburg FA, Mader U, Luster M, Reiners C. Histology does not influence prognosis in differentiated thyroid carcinoma when accounting for age, tumour diameter, invasive growth and metastases. Eur J Endocrinol. 2009;160:619–24.
4. Verburg FA, Mader U, Tanase K, Thies ED, Diessl S, Buck AK, Luster M, Reiners C. Life expectancy is reduced in differentiated thyroid cancer patients >= 45 years old with extensive local tumor invasion, lateral lymph node, or distant metastases at diagnosis and normal in all other DTC patients. J Clin Endocrinol Metab. 2013;98:172–80.
5. Tanase K, Thies ED, Mader U, Reiners C, Verburg FA. The TNM system (version 7) is the most accurate staging system for the prediction of loss of life expectancy in differentiated thyroid cancer. Clin Endocrinol. 2016;84(2):284–91.
6. Hedinger C, Williams ED, Sobin LH. Histological typing of thyroid tumours. No. 11 of international histologic classification of tumours. Berlin: Springer-Verlag; 1988.
7. Rosai J, Carcangiu ML, Delellis RA. Tumors of the thyroid gland. Atlas of tumor pathology, 3rd series. Fascicle 5. Armed Forces Institute of Pathology: Washington, D.C; 1992.
8. Kloos RT, Mazzaferri E. Thyroid carcinoma. In: Cooper DS, editor. Medical management of thyroid disease. New York: Marcel Dekker Inc.; 2001.
9. Shattuck TM, Westra WH, Ladenson PW, Arnold A. Independent clonal origins of distinct tumor foci in multifocal papillary thyroid carcinoma. N Engl J Med. 2005;352:2406–12.
10. Simpson WJ, Panzarella T, Carruthers JS, Gospodarowicz MK, Sutcliffe SB. Papillary and follicular thyroid cancer: impact of treatment

in 1578 patients. Int J Radiat Oncol Biol Phys. 1988;14:1063–75.

11. Hay ID, Bergstralh EJ, Grant CS, McIver B, Thompson GB, van Heerden JA, Goellner JR. Impact of primary surgery on outcome in 300 patients with pathologic tumor-node-metastasis stage III papillary thyroid carcinoma treated at one institution from 1940 through 1989. Surgery. 1999;126:1173–81.

12. Hay ID, Grant CS, Bergstralh EJ, Thompson GB, van Heerden JA, Goellner JR. Unilateral total lobectomy: is it sufficient surgical treatment for patients with AMES low-risk papillary thyroid carcinoma? Surgery. 1998;124:958–64.

13. Mazzaferri EL, Jhiang SM. Long-term impact of initial surgical and medical therapy on papillary and follicular thyroid cancer. Am J Med. 1994; 97:418–28.

14. Tsang RW, Brierley JD, Simpson WJ, Panzarella T, Gospodarowicz MK, Sutcliffe SB. The effects of surgery, radioiodine, and external radiation therapy on the clinical outcome of patients with differentiated thyroid carcinoma. Cancer. 1998;82:375–88.

15. Hay ID, Grant CS, Taylor WF, McConahey WM. Ipsilateral lobectomy versus bilateral lobar resection in papillary thyroid carcinoma: a retrospective analysis of surgical outcome using a novel prognostic scoring system. Surgery. 1987;102:1088–95.

16. Duren M, Yavuz N, Bukey Y, Ozyegin MA, Gundogdu S, Acbay O, Hatemi H, Uslu I, Onsel C, Aksoy F, Oz F, Unal G, Duren E. Impact of initial surgical treatment on survival of patients with differentiated thyroid cancer: experience of an endocrine surgery center in an iodine-deficient region. World J Surg. 2000;24:1290–4.

17. Pasieka JL, Thompson NW, McLeod MK, Burney RE, Macha M. The incidence of bilateral well-differentiated thyroid cancer found at completion thyroidectomy. World J Surg. 1992;16:711–6.

18. Cheah WK, Arici C, Ituarte PH, Siperstein AE, Duh QY, Clark OH. Complications of neck dissection for thyroid cancer. World J Surg. 2002;26:1013–6.

19. Thomusch O, Machens A, Sekulla C, Ukkat J, Lippert H, Gastinger I, Dralle H. Multivariate analysis of risk factors for postoperative complications in benign goiter surgery: prospective multicenter study in Germany. World J Surg. 2000;24:1335–41.

20. Dralle H, Sekulla C, Lorenz K, Brauckhoff M, Machens A. Intraoperative monitoring of the recurrent laryngeal nerve in thyroid surgery. World J Surg. 2008;32:1358–66.

21. Haugen BR, Alexander EK, Bible KC, Doherty GM, Mandel SJ, Nikiforov YE, Pacini F, Randolph GW, Sawka AM, Schlumberger M, Schuff KG, Sherman SI, Sosa JA, Steward DL, Tuttle RM, Wartofsky L. 2015 American thyroid association management guidelines for adult patients with thyroid nodules and differentiated thyroid cancer: The American thyroid association guidelines task force on thyroid nodules and differentiated thyroid cancer. Thyroid. 2016;26:1–133.

22. Diessl S, Holzberger B, Mader U, Grelle I, Smit JW, Buck AK, Reiners C, Verburg FA. Impact of moderate vs stringent TSH suppression on survival in advanced differentiated thyroid carcinoma. Clin Endocrinol. 2012;76:586–92.

23. Seidlin SM, Marinelli LD, Oshry E. Radioactive iodine therapy: effect on functioning metastases of adenocarcinoma of the thyroid. JAMA. 1946;132:838–47.

24. Eskandari S, Loo DD, Dai G, Levy O, Wright EM, Carrasco N. Thyroid Na+/I- symporter. Mechanism, stoichiometry, and specificity. J Biol Chem. 1997;272:27230–8.

25. Verburg FA, de Keizer B, Lips CJ, Zelissen PM, de Klerk JM. Prognostic significance of successful ablation with radioiodine of differentiated thyroid cancer patients. Eur J Endocrinol. 2005;152:33–7.

26. Mazzaferri EL, Kloos RT. Clinical review 128: current approaches to primary therapy for papillary and follicular thyroid cancer. J Clin Endocrinol Metab. 2001;86:1447–63.

27. Tubiana M, Schlumberger M, Rougier P, Laplanche A, Benhamou E, Gardet P, Caillou B, Travagli JP, Parmentier C. Long-term results and prognostic factors in patients with differentiated thyroid carcinoma. Cancer. 1985;55:794–804.

28. Utiger RD. Follow-up of patients with thyroid carcinoma. N Engl J Med. 1997;337:928–30.

29. Verburg FA, Dietlein M, Lassmann M, Luster M, Reiners C. Why radioiodine remnant ablation is right for most patients with differentiated thyroid carcinoma. Eur J Nucl Med Mol Imaging. 2009;36:343–6.

30. Sherman SI, Tielens ET, Sostre S, Wharam MD Jr, Ladenson PW. Clinical utility of posttreatment radioiodine scans in the management of patients with thyroid carcinoma. J Clin Endocrinol Metab. 1994;78:629–34.

31. Tenenbaum F, Corone C, Schlumberger M, Parmentier C. Thyroglobulin measurement and postablative iodine-131 total body scan after total thyroidectomy for differentiated thyroid carcinoma in patients with no evidence of disease. Eur J Cancer. 1996;32A:1262.

32. DeGroot LJ, Kaplan EL, Shukla MS, Salti G, Straus FH. Morbidity and mortality in follicular thyroid cancer. J Clin Endocrinol Metab. 1995;80:2946–53.

33. Samaan NA, Schultz PN, Hickey RC, Goepfert H, Haynie TP, Johnston DA, Ordonez NG. The results of various modalities of treatment of well differentiated thyroid carcinomas: a retrospective review of 1599 patients. J Clin Endocrinol Metab. 1992;75:714–20.

34. Cooper DS, Doherty GM, Haugen BR, Kloos RT, Lee SL, Mandel SJ, Mazzaferri EL, McIver B, Pacini F, Schlumberger M, Sherman SI, Steward DL, Tuttle RM. Revised American Thyroid Association management guidelines for patients with thyroid nodules and differentiated thyroid cancer. Thyroid. 2009;19:1167–214.

35. Pacini F, Schlumberger M, Dralle H, Elisei R, Smit JW, Wiersinga W. European consensus for the management of patients with differentiated thy-

roid carcinoma of the follicular epithelium. Eur J Endocrinol. 2006;154:787–803.

36. Luster M, Clarke SE, Dietlein M, Lassmann M, Lind P, Oyen WJ, Tennvall J, Bombardieri E. Guidelines for radioiodine therapy of differentiated thyroid cancer. Eur J Nucl Med Mol Imaging. 2008;35:1941–59.

37. Reiners C, Demidchik YE. Differentiated thyroid cancer in childhood: pathology, diagnosis, therapy. Pediatr Endocrinol Rev. 2003;1(Suppl 2):230–5.

38. Reiners C, Biko J, Haenscheid H, Hebestreit H, Kirinjuk S, Baranowski O, Marlowe RJ, Demidchik E, Drozd V, Demidchik Y. Twenty-five years after Chernobyl: outcome of radioiodine treatment in children and adolescents with very-high-risk radiation-induced differentiated thyroid carcinoma. J Clin Endocrinol Metab. 2013;98:3039–48.

39. Hanscheid H, Verburg FA, Biko J, Diessl S, Demidchik YE, Drozd V, Reiners C. Success of the postoperative 131I therapy in young Belarusian patients with differentiated thyroid cancer after Chernobyl depends on the radiation absorbed dose to the blood and the thyroglobulin level. Eur J Nucl Med Mol Imaging. 2011;38:1296–302.

40. Luster M, Felbinger R, Dietlein M, Reiners C. Thyroid hormone withdrawal in patients with differentiated thyroid carcinoma: a one hundred thirty-patient pilot survey on consequences of hypothyroidism and a pharmacoeconomic comparison to recombinant thyrotropin administration. Thyroid. 2005;15:1147–55.

41. Dow KH, Ferrell BR, Anello C. Quality-of-life changes in patients with thyroid cancer after withdrawal of thyroid hormone therapy. Thyroid. 1997;7:613–9.

42. Schroeder PR, Haugen BR, Pacini F, Reiners C, Schlumberger M, Sherman SI, Cooper DS, Schuff KG, Braverman LE, Skarulis MC, Davies TF, Mazzaferri EL, Daniels GH, Ross DS, Luster M, Samuels MH, Weintraub BD, Ridgway EC, Ladenson PW. A comparison of short-term changes in health-related quality of life in thyroid carcinoma patients undergoing diagnostic evaluation with recombinant human thyrotropin compared with thyroid hormone withdrawal. J Clin Endocrinol Metab. 2006;91:878–84.

43. Hanscheid H, Lassmann M, Luster M, Thomas SR, Pacini F, Ceccarelli C, Ladenson PW, Wahl RL, Schlumberger M, Ricard M, Driedger A, Kloos RT, Sherman SI, Haugen BR, Carriere V, Corone C, Reiners C. Iodine biokinetics and dosimetry in radioiodine therapy of thyroid cancer: procedures and results of a prospective international controlled study of ablation after rhTSH or hormone withdrawal. J Nucl Med. 2006;47:654.

44. Rosario PW, Borges MA, Purisch S. Preparation with recombinant human thyroid-stimulating hormone for thyroid remnant ablation with 131I is associated with lowered radiotoxicity. J Nucl Med. 2008;49:1776–82.

45. Frigo A, Dardano A, Danese E, Davi MV, Moghetti P, Colato C, Francia G, Bernardi F, Traino C, Monzani F, Ferdeghini M. Chromosome translocation frequency after radioiodine thyroid remnant ablation: a comparison between recombinant human thyrotropin stimulation and prolonged levothyroxine withdrawal. J Clin Endocrinol Metab. 2009;94:3472–6.

46. Haugen BR, Pacini F, Reiners C, Schlumberger M, Ladenson PW, Sherman SI, Cooper DS, Graham KE, Braverman LE, Skarulis MC, Davies TF, DeGroot LJ, Mazzaferri EL, Daniels GH, Ross DS, Luster M, Samuels MH, Becker DV, Maxon HR III, Cavalieri RR, Spencer CA, McEllin K, Weintraub BD, Ridgway EC. A comparison of recombinant human thyrotropin and thyroid hormone withdrawal for the detection of thyroid remnant or cancer. J Clin Endocrinol Metab. 1999;84:3877–85.

47. Borget I, Remy H, Chevalier J, Ricard M, Allyn M, Schlumberger M, De Pouvourville G. Length and cost of hospital stay of radioiodine ablation in thyroid cancer patients: comparison between preparation with thyroid hormone withdrawal and thyrogen. Eur J Nucl Med Mol Imaging. 2008;35:1457–63.

48. Borget I, Corone C, Nocaudie M, Allyn M, Iacobelli S, Schlumberger M, De Pouvourville G. Sick leave for follow-up control in thyroid cancer patients: comparison between stimulation with Thyrogen and thyroid hormone withdrawal. Eur J Endocrinol. 2007;156:531–8.

49. Bohuslavizki KH, Klutmann S, Jenicke L, Kroger S, Buchert R, Mester J, Clausen M. Salivary gland protection by S-2-(3-aminopropylamino)-ethylphosphorothioic acid (amifostine) in high-dose radioiodine treatment: results obtained in a rabbit animal model and in a double-blind multi-arm trial. Cancer Biother Radiopharm. 1999;14:337–47.

50. Kim SJ, Choi HY, Kim IJ, Kim YK, Jun S, Nam HY, Kim JS. Limited cytoprotective effects of amifostine in high-dose radioactive iodine 131-treated well-differentiated thyroid cancer patients: analysis of quantitative salivary scan. Thyroid. 2008;18:325–31.

51. Jentzen W, Schmitz J, Freudenberg L, Eising E, Hilbel T, Bockisch A, Stahl A. The influence of saliva flow stimulation on the absorbed radiation dose to the salivary glands during radioiodine therapy of thyroid cancer using 124I PET(/CT) imaging. Eur J Nucl Med Mol Imaging. 2010;37:2298–306.

52. Nakada K, Ishibashi T, Takei T, Hirata K, Shinohara K, Katoh S, Zhao S, Tamaki N, Noguchi Y, Noguchi S. Does lemon candy decrease salivary gland damage after radioiodine therapy for thyroid cancer? J Nucl Med. 2005;46:261–6.

53. Solans R, Bosch JA, Galofre P, Porta F, Rosello J, Selva-O'Callagan A, Vilardell M. Salivary and lacrimal gland dysfunction (sicca syndrome) after radioiodine therapy. J Nucl Med. 2001;42:738–43.

54. Seidlin SM, Siegal E, Yalow AA, Melamed S. Acute myeloid leukemia following prolonged iodine-131 therapy for metastatic thyroid carcinoma. Science. 1956;123:800–1.

55. Sawka AM, Thabane L, Parlea L, Ibrahim-Zada I, Tsang RW, Brierley JD, Straus S, Ezzat S, Goldstein DP. Second primary malignancy risk after radioactive

iodine treatment for thyroid cancer: a systematic review and meta-analysis. Thyroid. 2009;19:451–7.

56. Verkooijen RB, Smit JW, Romijn JA, Stokkel MP. The incidence of second primary tumors in thyroid cancer patients is increased, but not related to treatment of thyroid cancer. Eur J Endocrinol. 2006;155:801–6.

57. Benua RS, Cicale NR, Sonenberg M, Rawson RW. The relation of radioiodine dosimetry to results and complications in the treatment of metastatic thyroid cancer. AJR. 1962;1962:171–82.

58. Molinaro E, Leboeuf R, Shue B, Martorella AJ, Fleisher M, Larson S, Tuttle RM. Mild decreases in white blood cell and platelet counts are present one year after radioactive iodine remnant ablation. Thyroid. 2009;19:1035–41.

59. Verburg FA, Hanscheid H, Biko J, Hategan MC, Lassmann M, Kreissl MC, Reiners C, Luster M. Dosimetry-guided high-activity (131)I therapy in patients with advanced differentiated thyroid carcinoma: initial experience. Eur J Nucl Med Mol Imaging. 2010;37:896–903.

60. Molenaar RJ, Sidana S, Radivoyevitch T, Advani AS, Gerds AT, Carraway HE, Angelini D, Kalaycio M, Nazha A, Adelstein DJ, Nasr C, Maciejewski JP, Majhail NS, Sekeres MA, Mukherjee S. Risk of hematologic malignancies after radioiodine treatment of well-differentiated thyroid cancer. J Clin Oncol. 2018;36:1831–9.

61. Molenaar RJ, Pleyer C, Radivoyevitch T, Sidana S, Godley A, Advani AS, Gerds AT, Carraway HE, Kalaycio M, Nazha A, Adelstein DJ, Nasr C, Angelini D, Maciejewski JP, Majhail N, Sekeres MA, Mukherjee S. Risk of developing chronic myeloid neoplasms in well-differentiated thyroid cancer patients treated with radioactive iodine. Leukemia. 2018;32:952–9.

62. Piccardo A, Puntoni M, Verburg FA, Luster M, Giovanella L. Power of absolute values to avoid data misinterpretations: the case of radioiodine-induced leukemia and myelodysplasia. J Clin Oncol. 2018;36:1880–1.

63. Ain KB. Radioiodine-remnant ablation in low-risk differentiated thyroid cancer: pros. Endocrine. 2015;50:61–6.

64. Rosario PW, Barroso AL, Rezende LL, Padrao EL, Borges MA, Guimaraes VC, Purisch S. Testicular function after radioiodine therapy in patients with thyroid cancer. Thyroid. 2006;16:667–70.

65. Sawka AM, Lakra DC, Lea J, Alshehri B, Tsang RW, Brierley JD, Straus S, Thabane L, Gafni A, Ezzat S, George SR, Goldstein DP. A systematic review examining the effects of therapeutic radioactive iodine on ovarian function and future pregnancy in female thyroid cancer survivors. Clin Endocrinol. 2008;69:479–90.

66. Hebestreit H, Biko J, Drozd V, Demidchik Y, Burkhardt A, Trusen A, Beer M, Reiners C. Pulmonary fibrosis in youth treated with radioiodine for juvenile thyroid cancer and lung metastases after Chernobyl. Eur J Nucl Med Mol Imaging. 2011;38:1683–90.

Peptide Receptor Radionuclide Therapy for Neuroendocrine Tumors

4

Flavio Forrer

4.1 Introduction

Neuroendocrine tumors (NETs) are rare malignancies originating from neural crest cells. These cells belong to the amino precursor uptake and decarboxylation (APUD) system and can therefore accumulate and decarboxylate amine precursors. These cells can produce amines or hormones, such as histamine, serotonin, adrenaline, gastrin, and somatostatin (SST) that contribute to the onset of symptoms [1]. On the basis of symptoms NETs can be classified as functional (30–50%) and nonfunctional. Neural crest cells are characterized by the expression of neuroendocrine markers such as synaptophysin and chromogranin A [2].

Neuroendocrine cells are sparse throughout the whole body even though they are mainly concentrated in the gastrointestinal tract and the pancreas. Therefore NETs can originate in different parts of the body, mainly in the gastrointestinal tract (most frequently in jejunum, ileum, appendix and rectum) and in the endocrine pancreas (glucagonoma, insulinoma, vipoma, gastrinoma). However, NETs may originate in other anatomical sites as it is the case of bronchial carcinoid, neuroblastoma, and medullary thyroid cancer [3]. Secreting tumors may cause specific syndromes, including carcinoid syndrome, hypoglycemia, hyperglycemia, or Zollinger-Ellison syndrome. The carcinoid syndrome (diarrhea, skin-flushing, abdominal cramps, nausea, vomiting, and valvular heart disease) is the most common clinical syndrome and it is related to the production of serotonin and histamine. Many tumors may remain asymptomatic for many years. In 20–50% of cases, the primary origin cannot be identified and only liver or skeletal metastatic disease is detectable [1]. However, the sensitivity of detecting the primary increased significantly over the last years by improved imaging, in particular the use of Ga-68-labeled somatostatin analogues for PET-imaging [4].

More than 90% of NETs express somatostatin (SST) receptors [5]. SST is a peptide occurring in a 14-aminoacid isoform and in a 28-aminoacid isoform. SST is ubiquitous in the body, occurring prevalently in the central and peripheral nervous system, the gut, and the endocrine glands. SST exerts inhibitory effects on various hormonal systems and physiological functions, including cell growth. Five subtypes of the SST receptor (SST1–5) have been identified and cloned. There are five human SST receptor subtypes (SST1–SST5); all are expressed on tumors to some extent, but SST2 is by far the most abundant, whereas SST4 is seldomly found. In particular, in neuroendocrine tumors SST2 is by far the most often expressed receptor subtype. As typically SST2 is expressed homogeneously and in a high

F. Forrer (✉)
Clinics of Radiology and Nuclear Medicine,
Kantonsspital St. Gallen, St. Gallen, Switzerland
e-mail: flavio.forrer@kssg.ch

© Springer Nature Switzerland AG 2019
L. Giovanella (ed.), *Nuclear Medicine Therapy*, https://doi.org/10.1007/978-3-030-17494-1_4

density makes this receptor an excellent target for molecular radionuclide imaging and therapy [6].

4.2   Classification of Nets

Traditionally NETs were subdivided according to the section of the embryonal primitive gut from which they originated, i.e., foregut, midgut, and hindgut [7, 8].

However, nowadays a widely accepted, standardized classification system for GEP NETs with implications for clinical management as well as for prognosis as introduced by Rindi et al. using a TNM classification system analogous to the TNM classification used for other solid tumors should be used [9]. Grading schemes for neuroendocrine tumors (NETs) use mitotic count; the level of the nuclear protein Ki-67, which is associated with cellular proliferation; and assessment of necrosis. The World Health Organization (WHO) and the European Neuroendocrine Tumor Society (ENETS) both incorporate mitotic count and Ki-67 proliferation for the classification of gastroenteropancreatic NETs (GEP-NETs) [9, 10]. In the 2010 World Health Organization classification scheme NETs are classified as grade (G) 1 NETs, G2 NETs, neuroendocrine carcinomas (NEC G3), and mixed adenoneuroendocrine carcinomas (MANEC). Histologic grades are dependent on mitotic counts and the Ki-67 labeling index. In the most recently published 2017 revision for pancreatic neuroendocrine tumors NEC G3 are subdivided into neuroendocrine tumors NET G3 and neuroendocrine carcinoma NEC G3 [11].

4.3   Epidemiology

NETs are considered as rare tumors. However, the incidence is about up to five cases per 100,000 inhabitants, and since 5-year survival rates in patients with NETs, irrespective of stage of disease, are over 60% [8, 12–14], this results in a considerable prevalence. Non-localized disease at diagnosis occurs between 22% and 47% of patients [12, 13]. Moreover, the prevalence and incidence of NETs have increased substantially over the last three decades as awareness of the disease and diagnostic techniques have improved. This increase has been attributed primarily to the detection of clinically silent disease [1].

4.4   Diagnosis

The diagnosis of neuroendocrine tumor is typically achieved through the complementary use of laboratory and imaging techniques. Biochemical evaluation of secretory peptides and hormone should be performed. Computed tomography (CT), ultrasonography, angiography, and magnetic resonance imaging (MRI) are often performed subsequently. These techniques have good sensitivity but suffer from limited specificity.

Nuclear medicine techniques take advantage of the strong overexpression of SST receptors on NETs. As mentioned previously, the expression is vastly higher than on non-tumor tissues [5, 15]. SST2 receptors are the target of radioactive tracers used for somatostatin receptor scintigraphy (SRS) or positron emission tomography (PET)/CT. For this reason, these techniques have higher specificity than CT or MRI. For SRS several Indium-111 or Technetium-99m labeled compounds are available. [^{111}In-DTPA0]-octreotide (Octreoscan®), a specific radiolabeled agonist for SST receptors that binds preferably to SST2 receptors, is the best characterized compound. However, SRS suffers from sensitivity for lesions inferior to 1 cm also when tomographic acquisition (SPECT or SPECT/CT), rather than planar acquisition, is performed. Overall SRS has a sensitivity of approximately 57–77% for non-insulinomas and 25% for insulinomas [16].

Nowadays PET/CT can be regarded as the gold standard for well-differentiated neuroendocrine tumors. DOTA peptides labeled with [^{68}Ga] are most frequently used. These include [^{68}Ga]DOTATOC, [^{68}Ga]DOTANOC, and [^{68}Ga]DOTATATE [17]. All DOTA peptides bind to SST2 and with varying affinity to SST5 receptors as well. An example of [^{68}Ga]DOTATATE PET/CT of a patient suffering from a metastatic NET G1 of the small bowel is shown in Fig. 4.1.

Using another mechanism of accumulation 3,4-dihydroxy-6-18F-fluoro-L-phenylalanine

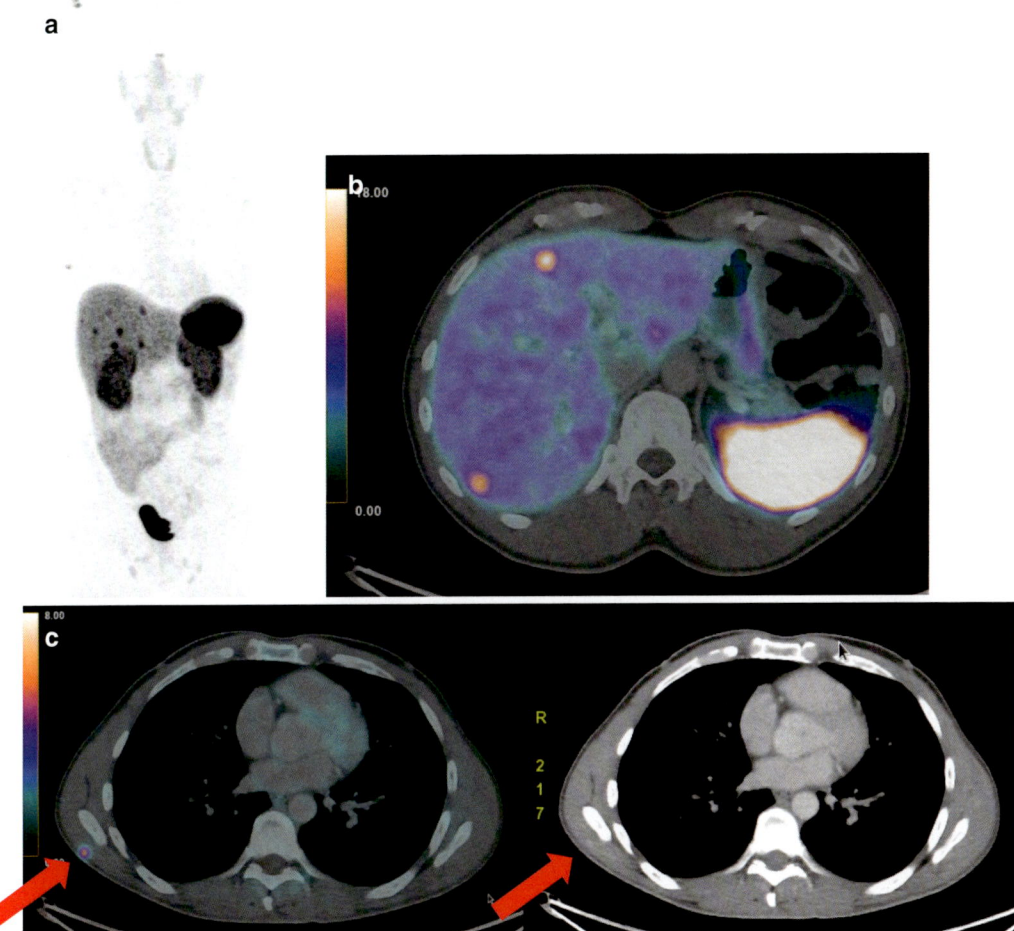

Fig. 4.1 ^{68}Ga-DOTATATE PET/CT of a patient with metastatic NET G1 of the small bowel. Panel (**a**) shows the maximum intensity projection (MIP) data. There is evidence of several liver metastases as well as of a focus on right thoracic side. Physiological uptake is seen in the pituitary gland, in the salivary glands, in the thyroid, in the liver, in the spleen, in the adrenals, and in the gall bladder. Additionally there is unspecific uptake in the bowel. Inguinal there is evidence of uptake in inflammatory lymph nodes. Panel (**b**) is a representative axial slice of the combined PET/CT through the abdomen. Intense focal uptake can be seen in two liver metastases in segment 4a and 7. High, physiological uptake is seen in the spleen. A soft tissue metastases in the right teres major muscle is presented in Panel (**c**). This lesion was diagnosed on the PET scan. Only retrospectively a corresponding focal contrast media accumulation was seen on the CT scan

(^{18}F-DOPA), an aromatic amino acid that is being trapped within neurotransmitter vesicles of NETs, can be used for diagnosis and staging as well with high sensitivity and specificity. However, in contrast to the SST binding compounds ^{18}F-DOPA is not suitable to select patients for radiopeptide therapy [18].

However, imaging can only provide localization of tumor lesions and demonstrate the presence of SST. Therefore, ultimate diagnosis requires histological demonstration of NETs after surgery or biopsy [11].

4.5   Therapy (Except Peptide Receptor Radionuclide Therapy)

Treatment is typically individualized and based on tumor stage, tumor burden, and symptoms [19–24]. The best therapeutic choice for individual patients will depend on whether the main aim of treatment is to slow tumor growth, to ameliorate symptoms by inhibition of the secretion of bioactive agents, or cure. An additional difficulty lies in the fact that there are no well-defined criteria to anticipate which tumors will respond to a particular modality or to assess rigorously therapeutic efficacy.

Surgery is essential for many patients with NETs. In patients with limited disease burden, surgery represents the primary method of cure [25]. For patients with advanced disease, cytoreductive surgery should be considered to increase the quality of life. The major limit to surgery is that more than 80% of patients have lymph node or liver metastases at the time of diagnosis [8, 26]. Therapy with SST analogs, such as octreotide and lanreotide, reduced amine production in functionally active NETs. SST analogues were shown to significantly lengthen time to tumor progression compared with placebo in patients with functionally active and inactive metastatic midgut NETs and are considered to be the first-line therapy in metastatic, well-differentiated tumors that cannot be cured by surgery [27]. The most effective and patient-friendly drugs are represented by long-acting octreotide acetate (Sandostatin LAR®) and lanreotide autogel (Somatuline®). SST analogues have a wide therapeutic range and are apparently free from major side effects. Minor gastrointestinal side effects are generally reported [27, 28].

Interferon-α may also be used for therapeutic purposes. However, side effects are prominent for interferon-α, which limits its clinical use. A randomized study using lanreotide alone or in combination with interferon-α reported a 5% partial response rate and a 25% stable disease rate over 12 months [29, 30].

Chemotherapy is performed using several drugs, including streptozotocin in combination with fluorouracil or doxorubicin, cisplatin and etoposide, and dacarbazine. Recently, some new chemotherapeutic agents have come into use, such as temozolomide, oxaliplatin, and capecitabine [31]. Chemotherapy has been recommended only for patients with poorly differentiated or rapidly progressing NETs or for patients that do not respond to SST analogues or interferon-α. With reference to histological types, chemotherapy is indicated especially in patients with pancreatic NETs, where it was shown effective in significantly reducing the tumor load [32].

In the last years, the efficacy of molecular targeting therapies for the therapy of NETs has been investigated. These treatments include angiogenesis inhibitors, single or multiple tyrosine kinase inhibitors, and the SST analogue pasireotide. The drugs with the highest evidence of efficacy are sunitinib and everolimus (RAD-001). Both lead to extension of progression-free survival (PFS) of patients with advanced pancreatic NET. For everolimus, an mTOR inhibitor, there is evidence of efficacy in controlling NET arising from other sites associated with the carcinoid syndrome [33]. The most developed antiangiogenic drugs are sunitinib and the anti-VEGF antibody bevacizumab. In a phase II study bevacizumab in combination with octreotide LAR led to partial tumor remission in 18% of patients and stable disease in 77% [34]. An international phase III study of sunitinib versus placebo in patients with progressive, well-differentiated endocrine pancreatic tumor was interrupted prematurely due to the striking superiority of sunitinib evident by a PFS of 11.1 vs. 5.5 months [35]. The objective remission rate was less than 10%. The drug is approved by the US FDA and the European Medicines Agency for the treatment of advanced and progressive well-differentiated pancreatic NETs. Everolimus has been studied in more than 1000 patients with NET and has been included in several clinical trials (RADIANT-1, RADIANT-2, RADIANT-3 trials, RAMSETE trial). Antitumor activity of everolimus has been confirmed in RADIANT-1 in patients with progressive metastatic pancreatic NETs after failure of at least one line of cytotoxic chemotherapy. The trial studied 160 patients divided into two groups with or without monthly intramuscular octreotide acetate therapy. The combination therapy showed significantly longer PFS (16.7 vs. 9.7 months) [36]. The efficacy of everolimus has been confirmed in a large international placebo-controlled trial, including 410 patients with progressive pancreatic NET (RADIANT-3) [37]. Everolimus significantly reduced the risk of disease progression and led to a prolongation of

PFS by 6.4 months (11 vs. 4.6 months) compared to placebo. Objective tumor response was low (4.8% partial remissions). Disease control rate (partial response + stable disease) was, however, higher with everolimus than with placebo with best supportive care (77.7% vs. 52.7%). Side effects were rarely grade 3 or 4; the most frequently reported side effects included stomatitis, anemia, and hyperglycemia.

Pain control in patients with NET is important when treating such patients. Pain therapy follows the general principles in oncology [38].

4.6 Peptide Receptor Radionuclide Therapy

Peptide receptor radionuclide therapy (PRRT) is another very attractive option for patients with metastatic NETs. Typically patients with progressive disease or symptomatic disease in whom surgery is no longer feasible are regarded as suitable candidates for this treatment modality [39]. PRRT is attractive because it is a systemic therapy that targets all SST-positive lesions, i.e., the primary tumor as well as distant metastases, and it is generally well tolerated by the patients.

Careful selection of patients is necessary to optimize the effects and minimize the potential side effects of PPRT. PRRT is indicated only in patients with histologically documented inoperable disease. The primary selection criterion is evidence of SST2 receptors overexpression by SST receptor imaging, either conventionally or by PET/CT with ^{68}Ga-labeled peptides. The intensity of tumor uptake must be equal or higher than in normal liver [40]. Traditionally, patients with evidence of progression of disease on CT or SRS have been referred to SRS. More recent data showed that the efficacy of therapy is greater in patients with stable disease than in patients with progressive disease [41–44], which indicated that patients with stable disease should also be considered for PRRT. Life expectancy greater than 3 months is a further requirement for treatment. Beside these selection criteria there is a number of contraindications which have to be respected:

4.6.1 Contraindications

All contraindications must be considered in the context of the other therapeutic options available, the patient's life expectancy, and whether the intent of treatment is symptom palliation or oncological control. Most are relative rather than absolute contraindications.

Pregnancy or ongoing lactation is regarded as an absolute contraindication. With regard to the health status severe hepatic impairment indicating biosynthetic liver failure (i.e., total bilirubin >3 upper limit of normal or both an albumin <25 g/L and prothrombin time increased >1.5 upper limit of normal) and severe cardiac impairment (New York Heart Association grade III or IV) are considered as absolute contraindications.

In the individual patient's context relative contraindications are:

- Significant sites of active disease as determined by unequivocal contrast-enhancing lesions on CT or MRI that lack SSTR expression, which can be confirmed by 18 F-FDG PET/CT if available (use of concomitant chemotherapy may be an option in such cases).
- Moderate to severe renal impairment (i.e., creatinine clearance <50 mL/min) patients on dialysis can be treated with a reduced administered activity to account for lack of urinary excretion with dialysis delayed for 24 h after treatment, subject to consultation with the managing nephrology team.
- Impaired hematological function, i.e., Hb <5 mmol/L (8 g/dL); platelets <75. 10 9/L; white blood cell count <2. 10 9/L$.
- Moderate to severe right heart valvular disease (valve replacement is strongly encouraged prior to PRRT; in such cases, please refer to the guidelines for the management of carcinoid heart disease).

Prior to PRRT and before each therapy cycle the following laboratory tests are required:

- Hematology: hemoglobin, white blood cell count plus differential, platelet number.

- Kidney function: creatinine and urea with formal creatinine clearance if abnormal.
- Liver function: bilirubin, albumin, ALP, GGT, ALT, AST, INR.
- Electrolytes: serum potassium and corrected serum calcium.
- LDH.

Additionally it is recommended to monitor Chromogranin A and other secretory products including specific hormones, if elevated at baseline.

4.6.2 Radiopharmaceuticals

There are different radiopharmaceuticals that may be used for PRRT. However, ^{177}Lu-DOTATATE ([^{177}Lu-DOTA^0,Tyr^3,Thr^8]-octreotide or [^{177}Lu-DOTA^0,Tyr^3]-octreotate) is the only FDA-approved compound for therapeutic purposes.

In general, each radiopharmaceutical that can be used for PRRT is composed by a peptide, which binds to the biological target (SST receptor), an isotope, that delivers the radioactivity to the tissue, and by a bifunctional chelator that is being used to connect the radioactive isotope and the peptide by making a stable complex between these molecules. In vitro studies showed that following the binding with an agonist, the SST receptor undergoes internalization. Internalization occurs as fast as within 3 min, is extremely efficient (most of the cell surface receptors are found in endosome-like structures), and is reversible (24 h after the receptors are again found at the cell surface) [45]. Following internalization, the radioactive peptide is trapped in the cell and exerts cytotoxic damages. SST2 receptor antagonists do not induce internalization. However, some recently published studies indicate that the tumor-to-background ratio might be even higher when using antagonists [46]. Theoretically this should result in a higher tumor absorbed dose without identical or even reduced toxicity. However, prospective or comparative studies are still lacking.

The first radiopharmaceutical used in peptide receptor radionuclide therapy (PRRT) was [^{111}In-DTPA^0]-octreotide. This peptide has been used since the 1980s for NET diagnosis and staging through SRS. [^{111}In-DTPA^0]-octreotide was used for therapy purpose with activities between 10 and 160 GBq, sizably higher than the activity (185–222 MBq) used for diagnostic purposes [47]. The rational for its use was represented by the fact that, in addition to the gamma-radiation, which makes ^{111}In suitable for imaging with a gamma-camera, ^{111}In emits Auger electrons. Auger electrons are low-energy electrons with a very short tissue penetration range of 0.02–10 μm. Auger electrons have a cytotoxic potential that requires close proximity of the ^{111}In-labeled peptide within the nucleus by interacting with the DNA after receptor internalization [48, 49].

Although Auger electrons do not display optimal therapeutic characteristics, [^{111}In-DTPA^0]-octreotide was chosen because at that time no other chelated SST analogue was available and DTPA itself was not a suitable chelator for the β-emitting radionuclides. Compared to other SST-analogues [^{111}In-DTPA^0]-octreotide has only a moderate affinity for SST2 receptors. An overview of the different affinity profiles is given in Table 4.1.

Over time other peptides with higher affinity towards SST receptors were synthesized and used in PRRT. The peptides include [Tyr3-octreotate] and lanreotide. A major breakthrough was achieved by the conjugation of SST-analogues with the chelator DOTA (1,4,7,10-tetraazacyclododecane-1,4,7,10-tetraacetic acid). DOTA has, in comparison to DTPA, better characteristics to stably bind beta (β-) emitting nuclides (^{90}Y and ^{177}Lu) as well as for positron (β+) emitting nuclides, and permits the use of such nuclides for therapy and imaging purposes [50, 51]. The available peptides have different affinities towards the various SST receptors. The affinity of a compound is significantly affected not only by the chelator but also by the radionuclide bound [52, 53]. The physical characteristics of the different radionuclides used in PRRT are presented in Table 4.2.

Table 4.1 Affinity profiles (IC 50) for human sst_1–sst_5 receptors of a series of somatostatin analogues

Peptide	sst_1	sst_2	sst_3	sst_4	sst_5
Somatostatin-28	5.2 ± 0.3 (19)	2.7 ± 0.3 (19)	7.7 ± 0.9 (15)	5.6 ± 0.4 (19)	4.0 ± 0.3 (19)
Octreotide	>10,000 (5)	2.0 ± 0.7 (5)	187 ± 55 (3)	>1000 (4)	22 ± 6 (5)
DTPA-octreotide	>10,000 (6)	12 ± 2 (5)	376 ± 84 (5)	>1000 (5)	299 ± 50 (6)
In-DTPA-octreotide	>10,000 (5)	22 ± 3.6 (5)	182 ± 13 (5)	>1000 (5)	237 ± 52 (5)
DOTA-TOC	>10,000 (7)	14 ± 2.6 (6)	880 ± 324 (4)	>1000 (6)	393 ± 84 (6)
Y-DOTA-TOC	>10,000 (4)	11 ± 1.7 (6)	389 ± 135 (5)	>10,000 (5)	114 ± 29(5)
DOTA-LAN	>10,000 (7)	26 ± 3.4 (6)	771 ± 229 (6)	>10,000 (4)	73 ± 12 (6)
Y-DOTA-LAN	>10,000 (3)	23 ± 5 (4)	290 ± 105 (4)	>10,000 (4)	16 ± 3.4 (4)
DOTA-OC	>10,000 (3)	14 ± 3 (4)	27 ± 9 (4)	>1000 (4)	103 ± 39 (3)
Y-DOTA-OC	>10,000 (5)	20 ± 2 (5)	27 ± 8 (5)	>10,000 (4)	57 ± 22 (4)
Ga-DOTA-TOC	>10,000 (6)	2.5 ± 0.5 (7)	613 ± 140 (7)	>1000 (6)	73 ± 21 (6)
Ga-DOTA-OC	>10,000 (3)	7.3 ± 1.9 (4)	120 ± 45 (4)	>1000 (3)	60 ± 14 (4)
DTPA-[Tyr^3]-octreotate	>10,000 (4)	3.9 ± 1 (4)	>10,000 (4)	>1000 (4)	>1000 (4)
DOTA-[Tyr^3]-octreotate	>10,000 (3)	1.5 ± 0.4 (3)	>1000 (3)	453 ± 176 (3)	547 ± 160 (3)
In-DTPA-[Tyr^3]-octreotate	>10,000 (3)	1.3 ± 0.2 (3)	>10,000 (3)	433 ± 16 (3)	>1000 (3)
Y-DOTA-[Tyr^3]-octreotate	>10,000 (3)	1.6 ± 0.4 (3)	>1000 (3)	523 ± 239 (3)	187 ± 50 (3)
Ga-DOTA-[Tyr^3]-octreotate	>10,000 (3)	0.2 ± 0.04 (3)	>1000 (3)	300 ± 140 (3)	377 ± 18 (3)

All values are IC 50 ± SEM in nM. The number of experiments is in parentheses
Reported after Reubi et al. [53]

Table 4.2 Physical properties of the most common radionuclides used in PRRT

Isotope	Half-life (d)	Decay mode	Energy	Range (max)
^{111}In	2.81	Auger	0.5–25 keV	10 μm
		γ	$E\gamma$: 0.173 MeV (87%), 0.247 MeV (94%)	
^{90}Y	2.67	β-	E_{max}: 2.28 MeV E_{mean}: 0.935 MeV	R_{max}: 11.3 mm R_{mean}: 4.1 mm
^{177}Lu	6.71	β-	E_{max}: 0.497 MeV E_{max}: 0.149 MeV	R_{max}: 2 mm R_{mean}: 0.5 mm
		γ	$E\gamma$: 0.113 MeV (6%), 0.208 MeV (11%)	

4.6.3   Studies Using [^{111}In-DTPA^0] octreotide

[^{111}In-DTPA^0]octreotide, developed initially for diagnosis [54], was the first radiolabeled SST analogue used for PRRT in cumulative activities ranging from 3.1 to 160 GBq [55–59]. Treatment with high activities often led to symptomatic relief; however, tumor shrinkage was rarely achieved and the number of objective responses was low. The first clinical trial of [^{111}In-DTPA^0] octreotide for treatment of NETs was performed by Krenning et al. in the Netherlands in 1994. Preliminary data from this study demonstrated the safety of repeated treatments with 333–666 MBq of [^{111}In-DTPA^0]octreotide administered every 3 weeks for 10 cycles. Tumor response correlated with receptor expression [57]. Valkema et al. in the Rotterdam study treated 50 patients with different histological NETs with cumulative activities of at least 20 GBq up to 160 GBq. PR was detected in 2% of patients, MR in 15% of patients, and stabilization of previously progressive tumors in 34% of patients [56].

In the New Orleans study Anthony et al. reported objective partial radiographic responses in 2/26 (8%) patients with metastatic NETs treated with [^{111}In-DTPA^0]octreotide and total cumulative activities of about 2 GBq. CT signs of partial tumor necrosis were detected in 7/26 (27%) patients. Moreover, they reported a median survival of 18 months. This value was sizably longer than the expected survival based on data obtained from historical controls treated with nonradioactive octreotide, indicating that treatment with ^{111}In-pentetreotide might prolong survival in GEP NETs [58].

The most common toxicity was due to bone marrow suppression. In the study by Valkema et al. serious side effects consisted of leukemia and myelodysplastic syndrome in 3/50 (6%) patients who had been treated with total cumulative activities of >3.7 GBq (and estimated bone marrow radiation doses of more than 3 Gy). One of these patients had also been treated with chemotherapy, which may have contributed to or caused this complication [56]. Anthony et al. reported renal insufficiency in one patient, which was probably not treatment-related, but due to preexistent retroperitoneal fibrosis. Transient liver toxicity was observed in three patients with widespread liver metastases [58].

In another study that was published some years later in NET patients treated with up to 38 GBq in two treatment cycles 53% of patients had grade I or II hematological toxicities, and 3% of patients had grade III thrombocytopenia. One patient (3%) had grade II liver toxicity, which appeared 4 weeks after therapy and resolved in the following week. No patient had renal toxicity. The toxicity profile of ^{111}In-pentetreotide was encouraging as the maximum tolerated dose was not achieved in any previously published studies, and it is possible that larger quantities of radioactivity can be administered safely [59].

Overall the results obtained with [^{111}In-DTPA^0] octreotide were encouraging, especially when seen in the context of the results that can be achieved with other therapy modalities like chemotherapy [60]. Nevertheless, it appeared that the antitumor effect of [^{111}In-DTPA^0]octreotide is not ideal for macroscopic tumors.

4.6.4 Studies Using [^{90}Y-DOTA^0,Tyr^3] octreotide (^{90}Y-DOTATOC), [^{90}Y-DOTA]lanreotide and [^{90}Y-DOTA^0,Tyr^3]octreotate

In order to improve the antitumor effect, subsequent studies were performed with ^{90}Y-labeled SST analogues. With the introduction of ^{90}Y the need of a new chelator arose since it cannot be bound in a sufficient stable way by DTPA [61]. ^{90}Y as well as ^{177}Lu are "bone seekers," i.e., free radionuclides would accumulate in the bone which consecutively would lead to a high absorbed dose to the bone marrow. DOTA is the most frequently used chelator in PRRT. DOTA has the ability to bind ^{90}Y as well as ^{177}Lu stably under various conditions [62].

The very first report on PRRT using ^{90}Y-DOTATOC was published in 1997 by the group at Basel University [63]. Biodistribution and clearance of ^{90}Y-DOTATOC were superior to [^{111}In-DTPA^0]octreotide. The kidney-to-tumor ratio was 1.9 times lower for ^{90}Y-DOTATOC than for [^{111}In-DTPA^0]octreotide. One of the three treated patients received therapeutic activities (3 GBq) of ^{90}Y-DOTATOC. Tumor progression was stopped in this patient as shown by follow-up diagnostic studies with [^{111}In-DTPA^0]octreotide. The patient also benefited clinically from the therapy as lower back and abdominal pain disappeared. These results were considered particularly promising considering that this patient had rapidly progressing liver and skeletal metastatic disease unresponsive to chemotherapy [63]. One year later the same group reported the results obtained in a larger sample of 10 patients. Overall 50% of patients experienced a PR and 50% experienced a SD [64].

The first study in a large population was published in 1999 [65]. Otte et al. treated 29 patients with escalating activities of ^{90}Y-DOTATOC in an interval of 6 weeks. Patients received a mean cumulative activity of 6.1 GBq/m2. They found that 69% of patients showed disease stabilization, 7% a partial remission, 14% a reduction of tumor mass < 50%, and 10% a progression of tumor growth [65].

Few years later, the group of Basel reported the results of their first phase-II study [66]. Forty-one patients with neuroendocrine GEP and bronchial tumors were included. 82% of the patients had therapy-resistant, progressive disease. The treatment consisted of four intravenous injections of a total of 6 GBq/m2 ^{90}Y-DOTATOC, administered at intervals of six weeks. The overall response rate was 24%. The response rate was higher (36%) in patients with endocrine pancreatic tumors. CR was found in 2%, PR in 22%, MR in 12%, SD in 49%, and PD in 15%. The median follow-up was 15 months. The survival at two years was 76% (95% confidence interval was 60%–92%). Eighty-three percent of the patients suffering from the malignant carcinoid syndrome achieved a significant reduction of symptoms. A reduction of pain score was observed in all patients taking morphine [66]. The OR in a following study with different patients was 23% [67]. Similar results were found in a more extensive study including 116 patients, who were treated with 6.0–7.4 MBq/m2 body surface (CR = 4%, PR = 23%, SD = 62% and PD = 11%) [68].

The research group from the European Cancer Institute in Milano used a higher range of cumulated activity (5.9 to 11.0 GBq in 2 cycles) in 21 patients with NETs, achieving an OR of 29%. All patients received amino acid infusion [69]. In a subsequent report extended to 141 patients with various SST-positive tumors, an OR of 26% (CR = 4%, PR = 22%) and a SD of 56% was reported. Interestingly, the favorable response rates were higher in patients that presented with stable disease before therapy (OR = 32%, SD = 64%) than in patients that were already progressive before therapy (OR = 23%, SD = 53%) [42].

Long-term follow-up and survival data for ^{90}Y-DOTATOC were published by Valkema et al. from the group at the University of Rotterdam [43]. In this study 58 patients were treated with 1.7–32.8 GBq of 90Y-DOTATOC. The response rates were comparable to other studies using 90Y-labeled SST analogues, but in addition a significant longer overall survival was shown compared to a group of historical controls treated with [^{111}In-DTPA^0]octreotide (37 vs. 12.0 months, respectively). Interestingly, overall survival was significantly better in patients who had SD at baseline vs. patients who had PD at baseline, in patients without liver metastases vs. patients with liver metastases, and in patients with high Karnofsky performance score vs. patients with low Karnofsky performance score.

The same group evaluated 42 patients with NETs within a phase I protocol [70]. In 32 patients who were given the planned activity, 3 patients had PR, 3 patients had MR, 17 had SD, and 9 had PD.

Chelated lanreotide, another SST analogue, labeled with ^{111}In for diagnostic purposes and with ^{90}Y for therapeutic use, has been advocated because of its better binding than [^{111}In-DTPA^0] octreotide to the SST receptor subtypes 3 and 4 [71]. This claim can be questioned [53]. Although this compound has been used to treat patients with GEP tumors, it shows poorer affinity than either DOTATOC or DOTATATE for SST2 receptors, which are predominantly overexpressed in GEP tumors.

^{90}Y-lanreotide was investigated in a European multicenter trial (MAURITIUS), in 154 patients administered with cumulative treatment activities ranging from 1.9 to 8.6 GBq of ^{90}Y-DOTA-lanreotide. Therapy entry criterion was progressive disease at the time of planned therapy. Preliminary treatment results in 154 patients indicated SD in 41% (63 of 154) of patients and PR in 14% (22 of 154) of tumor patients. No severe acute or chronic hematological toxicity, change in renal or liver function parameters caused by ^{90}Y-DOTA-lanreotide treatment were reported [71].

Cwikla reported on the effect of ^{90}Y-DOTATATE treatment in 60 patients with histologically proven GEP NETs [72]. Clinical responses were assessed 6 weeks after completing therapy and then after each of the 3- to 6-month intervals. Patients were treated with up to a cumulative activity of 15.2 GBq. At 6 months after final treatment, radiological PR was observed in 13 patients (23%), and the remaining patients had SD. Median progression-free survival (PFS) was 17 months, while the median overall survival (OS) was 22 months. In patients with early PD, the PFS was 4.5 and OS 9.5 months, while in those with SD or PR, PFS and OS were 19.5 and 23.5 months, respectively.

In summary, OR rates in patients treated with ^{90}Y-DOTATOC, ^{90}Y-DOTATATE, and ^{90}Y-DOTA-lanreotide were in range between 6% and 37% despite differences in the protocols used. These results and the prolonged overall survival represent an improvement in therapeutic effectiveness compared to the studies with [^{111}In-DTPA^0]octreotide.

4.6.5 Studies Using [^{177}Lu-DOTA^0,Tyr^3]octreotate (^{177}Lu-DOTATATE) and [^{177}Lu-DOTA^0,Tyr^3] octreotide (^{177}Lu-DOTATOC)

In 2003, the first study with ^{177}Lu-DOTATATE was published [44]. In this study 35 patients with GEP NETs were treated with escalating dosages up to a final cumulative activity of 22.2–29.6 GBq. An OR of 38% was found. The effects of the therapy on tumor size were assessed in 34 patients. Three months after the last administration, CR was found in 1 patient (3%), PR in 12 (35%), SD in 14 (41%), and PD in 7 patients (21%), including three patients who died during the treatment period. Tumor response was positively correlated with a high uptake on the octreoscan, limited hepatic tumor mass, and a high Karnofsky Performance Score. No serious side effects were reported.

In a later evaluation 310 patients were treated with up to a cumulative activity of 27.8–29.6 GBq, usually in four treatment cycles, with treatment intervals of 6–10 weeks. Serious adverse events that were likely attributable to the treatment were myelodysplastic syndrome in three patients, and temporary, nonfatal, liver toxicity in two patients. Complete and partial tumor remissions occurred in 2% and 28% of 310 NETs patients, respectively. Minor tumor response occurred in 16% of patients. Thus, OR occurred in 46% of patients. Compared with historical controls, there was a survival benefit of 40–72 months from diagnosis [73].

4.6.6 The First Randomized Controlled Trial of PRRT: NETTER-1

The first results of the to date only reported randomized trial concerning the efficacy of PRRT have recently been reported [74].

The NETTER-1 trial involved a 1: 1 randomization of 229 patients with progressive metastatic small intestinal NET on 30 mg monthly Sandostatin LAR to either ^{177}Lu-DOTA-octreotate with continuing Sandostatin LAR at 30 mg per month or to dose escalation of Sandostatin LAR to 60 mg monthly. The PRRT protocol involved 4 cycles of 7.4 GBq (200 mCi) of ^{177}Lu-DOTAoctreotate at 8 weekly intervals. Most (77%) patients received all planned cycles of treatment. For the PRRT arm, a median PFS was not reached compared to 8.4 months ($p < 0.001$) for dose-escalated Sandostatin LAR. All predefined subanalysis groups had improved PFS with ^{177}Lu-DOTA-octreotate compared to controls. Although the relatively short duration of follow-up at the time of publication limited assessment of OS in either group, interim analysis indicated that the estimated risk of death was 60% lower in the ^{177}Lu-DOTA-octreotate group than in the control group (hazard ratio 0.40; $p = 0.004$). The objective response rate was 18 versus 3% ($p < 0.0004$). Grade 3 or 4 neutropenia, thrombocytopenia, and lymphopenia occurred in 1, 2, and 9% of patients in the PRRT arm versus none in controls. One case of MDS was attributed to PRRT.

The most commonly reported acute side effects of PRRT were nausea and vomiting. These occurred primarily during amino acid infusion given for renal protection and resolved with cessation of the infusion. In this trial, commercial amino acid solutions (Aminosyn II 10% [21.0 g of lysine and 20.4 g of arginine in 2 L of solution] or VAMIN-18 [18 g of lysine and 22.6 g of arginine in 2 L of solution]) were administered. These solutions are more concentrated than those used in most institutional trials, which typically include only lysine and arginine.

Use of anti-emetic medication was not reported but is an effective means to reduce these side effects. Although these results are entirely in keeping with other phase I–II institutional trials and retrospective analyses of single institutional experience, final analysis of the longer-term toxicity, quality of life, and patient outcome data are not yet available through peer-reviewed publication.

Some months later the same group proofed that in addition to improving progression-free survival, ^{177}Lu-Dotatate provides a significant quality-of-life-benefit for patients with progressive midgut NETs compared with high-dose octreotide [75].

4.6.7 Studies Combining Radionuclides and Utilizing Radiosensitizing Chemotherapy

Many trials mentioned above and other institutional series suggest that treatment with radio-labeled somatostatin analogues is an effective therapeutic modality in the management of patients with inoperable or metastasized NETs. However, a significant variability remains in the approach to delivering this therapy. While the NETTER-1 trial used a fixed administered activity of ^{177}Lu-DOTA-octreotate, others have used variable administered activities, different radionuclides, routes of administration, and intervals between treatments. Eligibility criteria have also varied. A variation in the treatment protocol has included the use of combinations of different radionuclides to optimize delivery to lesions of different sizes. For example, ^{90}Y has theoretical advantages for lager lesions with more heterogeneous uptake due to its long β-particle path length whereas ^{177}Lu is better suited to smaller lesions [76]. Accordingly, using these isotopes in combination might provide better radiation dose delivery across the range of lesion sizes that is often present in individual patients. Indeed, results of combination therapies are encouraging [77, 78]. Similarly, although most PRRT have involved intravenous administration, liver-dominant disease may benefit from hepatic arterial administration [79] but no prospective comparison studies are currently available.

While a standardized approach is likely to better meet the regulatory requirements for reimbursement, the need for a more individualized approach has also been argued [80]. This includes the potential use of PRRT in combination with other therapies in a manner analogous to chemoradiation, which is now widely used in the treatment of various solid tumors. Studies combining PRRT with radiosensitizing chemotherapy, which has been called peptide receptor chemoradionuclide therapy (PRCRT), have shown that this is feasible with minimal incremental toxicity. This approach has included studies with infusion of 5-fluorouracil or administration of its oral prodrug, capecitabine [81–84], and a further study using capecitabine and temozolomide [85].

While according to the data available safe and efficacious, there are currently no data confirming whether PRCRT is superior to PRRT. The rationale for combining chemotherapy with PRRT is strongest for higher-grade NEN. In lower-grade NETs, which would be expected to have longer survival independent of therapeutic effects, the potential benefits of chemotherapy need to be balanced against the risks of inducing MDS or leukemia, which may be more likely when an alkylating agent like temozolomide is used [86].

4.6.8 Re-treatment

In patients who responded to PRRT the question arises whether re-treatment is useful in case of relapse. The first study dealing with re-treatment in PRRT reported the results of using ^{177}Lu-DOTATOC in 27 patients after relapse from ^{90}Y-DOTATOC therapy. Inclusion criteria was that the patients achieved at least a SD after ^{90}Y-DOTATOC treatment and thereafter were progressive again. After restaging, PR in 2 patients, MR in 5 patients, SD in 12 patients, and PD in 8 patients was found. It was concluded that ^{177}Lu-DOTATOC therapy in patients with relapse after [90]YDOTATOC treatment is feasible, safe, and efficacious [87]. Frilling et al. treated with ^{177}Lu-DOTATOC 20 patients with metastatic non-resectable NETs refractory to ^{90}Y-treatment. In eight patients the treatment was repeated more than once. No serious adverse events were documented. After restaging, a PR was found in 5 patients, SD in 11 patients, and PD in 4 patients [88].

A study from the National Cancer Institute in Milano reported feasibility and utility of re-treatment with ^{177}Lu-DOTATATE in GEP-NENs relapsed after treatment with ^{90}Y-DOTATOC.

Twenty-six patients were enrolled and the disease control rate was found to be 84.6%. They concluded that patients with GEP-NEN who have previously responded to Y-PRRT are suitable candidates for Lu-PRRT re-treatment on progression [89].

4.6.9 Dosimetry

Radiation dosimetry aims at calculating the amount of radioactivity absorbed dose by tissues following PRRT. The absorbed radiation dose is expressed in grays (Gy), i.e., the amount of transferred energy in Joule per Kg. The rational of dosimetry stems from the assumption that patients should be treated with the highest possible activity that does not cause significant toxicity. The higher the absorbed dose to the tumor, the greater is the likelihood of a significant therapeutic effect. However, the dose must not be so high to induce clinically important organ toxicity. Individual patient dosimetry has the following goals: (1) to quantify minimum effective and maximum tolerated effective doses; (2) to establish a dose-response relation to predict tumor response and normal organ toxicity; and (3) to objectively compare the dose-response results of different radionuclide therapies [90].

Radiation dosimetry requires knowledge of the kinetics of the radiopharmaceutical in different body compartments so that a mathematical model may be developed relating the concentration of the tracer in tissue compartments to tissue absorbed dose. Several planar or tomographic acquisitions are performed starting from tracer injection to few days post injection and multiple blood and urine samples are obtained. Values of organ activity over times are interpolated and extrapolated to infinity to obtain a time-activity curve (TAC). The early (growing) part of the TAC is typically fitted using linear regression while the wash-out (descending) part is fitted using a mono- or bi-exponential function. Fitting provides measurement of the residence time of tracers in various organs. Residence times are input to software that uses the Medical Internal Radiation Dose (MIRD) formalism to calculate dosimetry estimates. Commercially available software such as MIRDOSE or OLINDA are provided with internal model about anatomy (standard man and woman) and radiopharmaceutical distribution (uniformity of uptake in source and target) [91].

Although these models are not necessarily valid in individual patients, they do provide a practical and standardized model for clinical end-users [90]. Dosimetric studies showed that the median absorbed dose was higher in responsive tumors than in nonresponsive tumors (230 Gy vs. 40 Gy, respectively); a linear relationship between absorbed dose and development of toxicity has not been observed [92]. Moreover, clinical trials evidenced large patient variability regarding target and nontarget uptake, and inhomogeneity of uptake within tumor sites [93, 94]. For these reasons and for the relative complexity in the execution of lengthy dosimetric studies, the clinical usefulness of personalized dosimetry has been debated and many institutions use fixed amount of radioactivity to all patients or activities based on kg or m^2 of body surface. It has been stated that "claims for specific dosimetry have to demonstrate that the frequency of excess toxicity and/or tumor underdosing significantly decreases" [95]. Dosimetry should provide a quantification procedure that is primarily of additional benefit over empirical, fixed dosing [90].

4.6.10 Dosimetry for ^{90}Y- and ^{177}Lu

The most commonly used ^{90}Y- and ^{177}Lu-labeled SST analogues concord on some essential aspect [96]: (1) the pharmacokinetics data show very fast blood clearance and urinary elimination; (2) the spleen, kidneys, and liver receive the highest absorbed dose; (3) kidneys and bone marrow are the major activity limiting organs for this treatment; and (4) there is a wide inter-patient variability of the absorbed dose. However, due to the physical characteristics of the radionuclides, the absorbed doses with ^{90}Y radiolabeled analogues are higher than those obtained with ^{177}Lu radiolabeled peptides, for the same injected activity. Issues affecting dosimetry studies are also different for different nuclides.

[177]Lu, in addition to beta particles, emits two distinct gamma photons (Table 4.2). Thus, for ^{177}Lu-labeled peptides, dosimetry and therapy may be performed at the same time (Fig. 4.2). In contrast ^{90}Y is a pure beta emitter and alternative strategies need to be adopted for external imaging such as the use of ^{111}In as surrogate [97]. Owing to the large availability, [^{111}In-DTPA[0]]-octreotide has been used as a surrogate of ^{90}Y-DOTATOC [92]. However, due to the different kinetics of the different radiolabeled conjugates chelators (DTPA vs. DOTA), the use of [^{111}In-DTPA0]-octreotide does not accurately reflect the distribution of ^{90}Y-DOTATOC [53].

[68]Ga-labeled peptides can also been used for diagnostic purposes. However, ^{68}Ga has a relatively short half-life (68 min) so that derivation of the late part of tissue TAC is not possible. Besides it is possible that ^{68}Ga peptides have different pharmacokinetics in comparison to [90]Y- or ^{177}Lu-labeled compounds [96].

Another option for performing ^{90}Y dosimetry is using Bremsstrahlung imaging [98]. The second modality developed relates to the use of time-of-flight PET/CT. The decay of ^{90}Y has a minor branch to the 0+ excited state, followed by an internal e+ e− creation and consequently photon annihilation. Using this approach the distribution of radioactivity following ^{90}Y-radioembolization was quantified. However, this approach is technologically challenging [99].

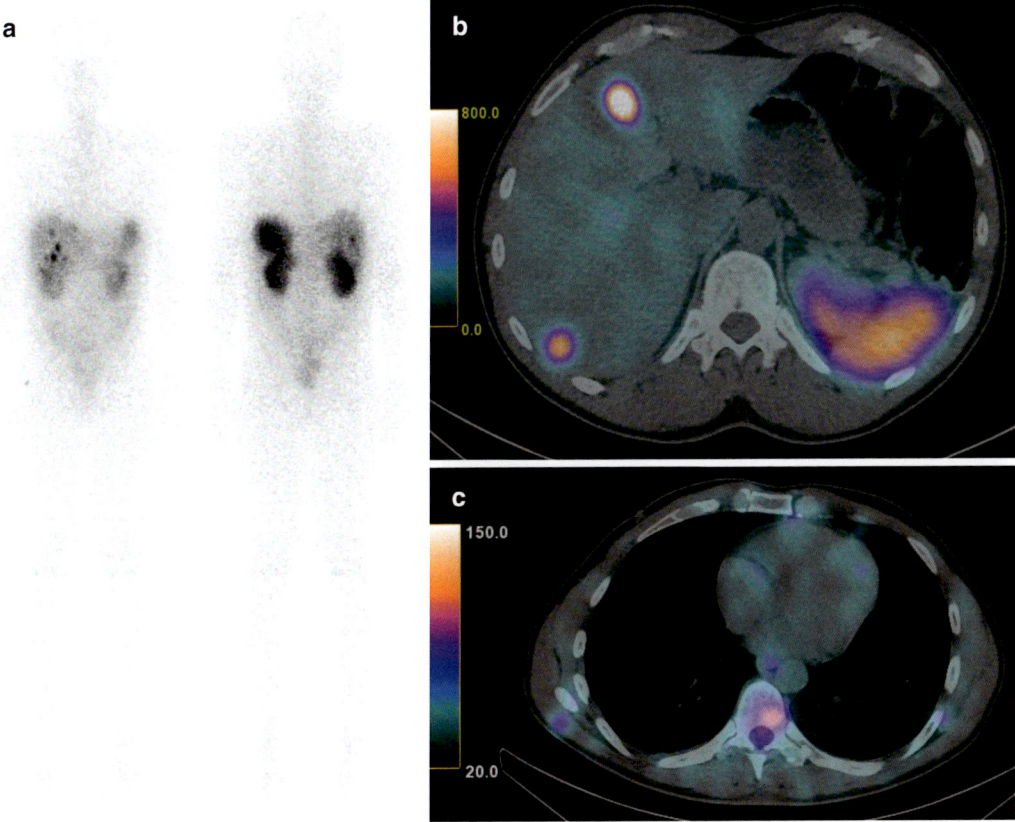

Fig. 4.2 Post-therapeutic planar whole body scan (panel **a**) and SPECT/CT (panel **b**) of the same patient that is presented in Fig. 4.1. The scans were acquired 24 h after the first injection of 7400 MBq ^{177}Lu-DOTATOC. There is evidence of high specific uptake in the known liver metastases corresponding well with the axial slice presented in Fig. 4.1. Only faint uptake can be seen in the soft tissue metastases (panel **c**)

4.6.11 Side Effects and Toxicity

Generally PRRT can be regarded as a relatively safe treatment and severe side effects are rare. Potential side effects may be predicted by the physiological distribution of radioactivity in PET/CT using DOTAT peptides. Physiological binding occurs in organs expressing SST2 receptors, such as the pituitary gland, the thyroid, the spleen, the adrenals, the kidneys, and the liver. In addition, the amount of radioactivity in the plasma is a significant source of exposure to bone marrow [100]. The side effects in PRRT can be divided into acute side effects and more delayed effects caused by radiation toxicity.

The acute effects occurring at the time of injection up to a few days after therapy include nausea, vomiting, and increased pain at tumor sites, symptoms that were reported after treatments with all radionuclides [58, 67, 74]. These side effects are generally mild, and can be prevented or reduced by anti-emetic treatment or steroids. The NETTER-1 trial reported nausea and vomiting in up to 59% in the radiopeptide arm. Abdominal pain was reported in 26% in the radiopeptide arm. However abdominal pain in 26% of the patients was found in the Sandostatin LAR arm as well [74]. Similar side effects are seen using ^{90}Y-DOTATATE [76]. In patients treated with ^{177}Lu-DOTATATE mild hair loss was reported in up to 60% of patients, however hair growth normalized at follow-up 3 to 6 months after the treatment [73].

Beside these minor side effects severe late toxicity may occur as a result of the radiation absorbed dose in healthy organs. The organs at risk are mainly the bone marrow, the kidneys, and to a lower extent the liver.

4.6.12 Renal Toxicity

The radiopeptides are filtered by the glomerulus. Although the major part of the radiopharmaceutical is excreted into the urine, peptides are partially taken up in proximal tubule cells by the multiligand scavenger receptor megalin and subsequently trapped into lysosomes leading to a considerable radiation to the kidneys [101–103]. The receptor involved in the renal uptake of radioactive peptides binds various structurally different proteins, including albumin and β_2-microglobulin. The localization of the radiopeptide in the kidney is not homogeneous, but it occurs predominantly in the cortex where it follows a striped pattern, with most of the radioactivity centered in the inner cortical zone [104]. This pattern of uptake results in different activity distributions for different radionuclides [105].

Bodei et al. assessed the role of clinical risk factors for the development of kidney toxicity in 28 patients receiving ^{90}Y-DOTATOC ($n = 23$) and ^{177}Lu-DOTATOC ($n = 5$) studied with a median follow-up of 28 months. Risk factors included hypertension, diabetes, renal morphological abnormalities, the use of radiological contrast medium and previous chemotherapy with nephrotoxic agents. The cumulative BED was higher in patients without risk factors (40 Gy) than in patients with risk factors (28 Gy). Risk factors were significantly more frequent in patients that developed increased creatinine levels in comparison to patients that did not develop nephrotoxicity [106]. Other factors that may increase the risk of nephrotoxicity are cumulative renal radiation dose, per cycle renal activity (i.e., therapy fractioning), kidney volume, and increasing age [92, 94, 107]. The damage to the kidney seems to be progressive and nephrotoxicity may appear as times goes on. Valkema et al. reported a decrease in creatinine clearance of 7.3% per year for ^{90}Y-DOTATOC and of 3.6% per year for ^{177}Lu-DOTATOC [107]. The increase in creatinine levels may occur even 1–2 years after the end of the therapy [106].

Several strategies may be adopted to reduce kidney toxicity. The clinically most relevant strategy is to interfere with the uptake of radiolabeled peptides. Basic amino acids, including arginine and lysine, bind to megalin via their cationic sites and competitively inhibit renal reabsorption of radioactive peptide used in PRRT. Therefore, basic amino acids are recommended to be used routinely to reduce renal uptake of radiolabeled peptides [108, 109]. The reduction in renal uptake induced by cationic amino acids ranges between

15% and 60% depending on the amount of amino acids being used and on the experimental design [69, 110, 111]. Amino acids are infused slowly over a 4–10 h period. However, amino acids have some disadvantages. For examples, they can induce nausea and vomiting, hyperkalemia, and arrhythmias [112, 113].

Other strategies have been investigated preclinically such as the use of the plasma expander gelofusine [114] or the use of the radioprotective drug amifostine [115]. However, the benefit for patients during PRRT remains to be proven and studies in patients are lacking.

In general, renal toxicity following PRRT seems to be a problem when using ^{90}Y as the therapeutic radionuclide. While in studies using ^{90}Y-DOTATOC the rate of severe and irreversible kidney toxicity (grade 4 & 5) was reported to be up to 9.2% after a median follow-up of 23 month [116], no grade 4 or 5 toxicity was reported in the NETTER-1 study after a median follow-up of 14 months [74].

Also no renal toxicity was reported after the therapeutic use of very high activities of [^{111}In-DTPA^0]octreotide [56]. These differences in renal toxicity occur although dosimetric analysis shows comparable absorbed doses to the kidney. The reason is most likely the heterogeneous dose distribution with significant differences between the various radionuclides [101]. The physical characteristics of the radionuclide have a significant impact on renal toxicity, i.e., Auger electrons emitted by ^{111}In and low-energy electrons emitted by ^{177}Lu have a short spatial range and do not reach the radiosensitive glomerulus.

For future calculations of the absorbed dose to normal organs and tumors these micro-dosimetric aspects are crucial to be taken into consideration.

4.6.13 Hematological Toxicity

With regard to hematological toxicity one needs to differentiate between early, transient toxicity and severe irreversible long-term toxicity such as a myelo-dysplastic syndrome (MDS). As MDS is typically late toxicity the reports are inconsistent. A range between 0.2% after therapy with ^{90}Y-DOTATOC [116] and 1.4% after treatment with ^{177}Lu-DOTATATE [117] is reported in literature. However, in particular when combining PRRT with chemotherapy the rate might be much higher [118].

Also high rate of MDS has been reported after the therapeutic use of [^{111}In-DTPA^0]-octreotide with MDS rates up to 6% [56]. Beside the limited efficacy this is another reason why [^{111}In-DTPA^0]-octreotide should not be used anymore for PRRT.

The MDS rate in the NETTER-1 trial, after the previously mentioned median follow-up of 14 months, was found to be 0.9%. However, as the typical time point of MDS onset is approximately 2 years, a somewhat higher rate must be expected [74].

Essentially all studies investigating PRRT report transient hematological toxicity. It appears that the absorbed radiation dose to the bone marrow is mainly caused by the circulation of the radioactivity in the blood. The most commonly adopted approach for calculation of bone marrow dosimetry is represented by the blood based approach, whereby it is assumed that there is no specific binding of the radiopeptide in the bone marrow and the unique source of radiation exposure is represented by the blood [100].

Severe hematological toxicity (grade 3 or 4 for hemoglobin, white blood cells and platelets) is reported in approximately 10–12% of the patients treated [73, 116, 117]. The NETTER-1 study reports transient lymphopenia grade 3 or 4 in 9% of the patients in the PRRT arm [74]. In contrast to renal toxicity which seems to be somewhat more pronounced when using ^{90}Y, no relevant difference between ^{90}Y and ^{177}Lu was found for hematological toxicity.

The likelihood of a severe toxicity increases with repeated cycles [44, 119].

In general, the decrease in blood count is transient. Blood transfusions were needed only occasionally and patients recovered fully. Bone marrow has been regarded as the dose-limiting organ in approximately 70% of patients treated with ^{177}Lu-DOTATATE [120].

With regard to dosimetric aspects it is generally accepted that in order to avoid bone marrow hypoplasia a maximum absorbed dose of 2 Gy should not be exceeded [44, 111]. Already back in 1962, in thyroid cancer patients treated with radioiodine, an absorbed dose of 2 Gy to the bone marrow resulted in a probability for developing leukemia of approximately 2% [121]. This seems to be very well in line with the results after PRRT.

Generally, the cause for myelodysplastic syndrome cases is difficult to be defined as many patients that are included into PRRT trials were pretreated with either chemotherapy or external beam radiation. In summary hematological toxicity following PRRT is frequent but generally mild and transient. Myelodysplastic syndrome may occur, even though the risk is low especially in the absence of previous chemotherapy and radiotherapy.

4.6.14 Liver Toxicity

Beside the fact that most patients who are treated with PRRT suffer from liver metastases, physiological uptake in normal liver tissue also occurs after administration of radiolabeled SST analogues. The sum of this physiological uptake and the dose to the normal liver deriving from the specific uptake in liver metastases can result in a considerable radiation absorbed dose to the liver [122]. However, since the tumor load in the liver shows high inter-patient variability, it is difficult to generalize about the radiation absorbed doses to the liver.

A significant increase in liver enzymes after the administration of radiopeptides was reported in several studies. Valkema et al. reported one transient grade 3 toxicity in a group of 60 patients treated with ^{90}Y-DOTATOC in a phase I study [43]. In another study, 15 patients with known liver metastases (of whom 12 had extensive liver involvement, defined as 25% or more) from NETs were treated with three cycles of 4.4 GBq each [123]. In four of these 15 patients, one or more of the three liver enzymes that were measured (serum aspartate aminotransferase, alanine aminotransferase and alkaline phosphatase) increased. Increase was defined as at least one grade, according to the WHO criteria, from baseline to final follow-up measurement (4–6 weeks post cycle 3). It was concluded that patients with diffuse SST-positive hepatic metastases could be treated with up to a cumulative administered

activity of (13.3 GBq of ^{90}Y-DOTATOC with only a small chance of developing mild acute or subacute hepatic injury.

In the group of patients treated with ^{177}Lu-DOTATATE, significantly increased liver function parameters (grade 4 liver toxicity) were evident in two patients after the first cycle of treatment [124]. A study focusing on hepatic toxicity found a relative risk of hepatotoxicity related to PRRT exposure in metastatic GEP-NET in 1.94% [125].

No hepatic toxicity is reported in the NETTER-1 trial.

In summary, liver toxicity is rare and if it occurs it is mostly mild and reversible. However, extensive liver metastases seem to be a risk factor for liver impairment after PRRT. In these patients it may be difficult to distinguish between real toxicity caused by radiation from effects by the metastases themselves.

4.6.15 Endocrine Toxicity

SST receptors are expressed by several glands, including the pituitary gland, thyroid, endocrine pancreas, and adrenal medullas. Thus, it is of interest to investigate whether PRRT is associated with significant endocrine toxicity. Teunissen et al. addressed this issue in 35 men and 21 females treated with 22.2–29.6 GBq of ^{177}Lu-octreotate in 3–4 cycles with 6–9 weeks interval and followed up for up to 24 months [126]. In 35 men, mean serum levels of inhibin B that is produced by the Sertoli cells of the testis were decreased at 3 months post-therapy and follicle-stimulating hormone (FSH) levels increased. These levels returned to near baseline levels after 24 months. Total testosterone and sex hormone binding globulin levels decreased. An increase of luteinizing hormone (LH) levels was found at 3 months of follow-up returning to baseline levels thereafter. In 21 postmenopausal women, a decrease in levels of FSH and LH was found. Of 66 patients, 2 developed persistent primary hypothyroidism. Before and after therapy adrenocorticotropic hormone stimulation test showed an adequate response of serum cortisol. Five patients developed elevated Hemoglobin A1C. These results indicate that ^{177}Lu-octreotate therapy induced transient inhibitory effects on spermatogenesis. In the long term, gonadotropin levels decreased significantly in postmenopausal women. Overall, PRRT with ^{177}Lu-octreotate can be regarded as a safe treatment modality with respect to short- and long-term endocrine function [126].

The NETTER-1 study as well as most of all the other studies cited above do not repost endocrine toxicity.

4.6.16 Factors Affecting the Response to Therapy

An important issue would be to determine negative and positive prognostic factors relevant for therapy response and survival. This would allow identifying patients susceptible to benefit from more intensive treatment schemes.

However, to date prognostic or predictive factors are still not well investigated and are often mixed up. For example, Brunner et al. demonstrated the SST2 expression to be an independent prognostic factor for NET patients [127] although it is most likely that a high SST2 expression is a predictive factor for a good response to PRRT as well [108].

The subgroup analysis in the NETTER-1 study showed consistent benefit for PRRT across major subgroups in comparison to the Sandostatin arm. This is a clear indication that the selection criteria used in this trial are when patients are useful.

The degree of liver involvement is inversely related to the chance of remission [128]. Poorer prognosis was also reported for patient having elevated alkaline phosphatase concentrations in serum [73, 129].

Poor performance status has been consistently associated with poor response to therapy and poor survival [43, 73].

4.6.17 Dedifferentiation and Glucose Metabolism

An interesting factor that was investigated by several groups is FDG uptake in ^{18}F-FDG-PET/CT. The uptake of FDG is usually poor in the majority of well-differentiated NET G1 and G2.

FDG-positive disease is found approximately in 40% of G1 patients and 70% of G2 patients [130]. In the same work the group found that FDG-uptake has a very high prognostic value in patients with NET. For prediction of OS of patients with NET the hazard ratio between patients with positive ^{18}F-FDG PET and negative ^{18}F-FDG PET was 10 and it exceeded the prognostic value of traditionally used parameters, such as Ki-67, Chromogranin A level, and the presence of liver metastases. Garin et al. showed in a prospective study including 38 patients that ^{18}F-FDG PET/CT identifies patients who have rapidly progressive NETs and that ^{18}F-FDG PET scan is an independent predictor of PFS [131]. Therefore, FDG imaging should be considered in NET patients beside the low sensitivity.

4.7   Conclusions

PRRT is an exciting, effective and safe treatment modality for patients with metastatic, inoperable, neuroendocrine tumors. So far it is mainly indicated for patients with NET G1 and NET G2. A high expression of somatostatin receptors demonstrated by imaging is an absolute prerequisite for this treatment.

Toxicity, when using ^{177}Lu labeled peptides, is mainly hematological and in an acceptable range. Severe irreversible toxicity is rare.

While two decades ago only very few centers could offer PRRT, the availability of PRRT will increase dramatically with the recent FDA-approval of ^{177}Lu-DOTATATE (Lutathera®). This will allow to conduce further clinical trials who will help us to answer some of the many questions that still remain to be answered in the context of NET and PRRT.

References

1. Modlin IM, Oberg K, Chung DC, et al. Gastroenteropancreatic neuroendocrine tumours. Lancet Oncol. 2008;9(1):61–72.
2. Wiedenmann B, John M, Ahnert-Hilger G, et al. Molecular and cell biological aspects of neuroendocrine tumors of the gastroenteropancreatic system. J Mol Med (Berl). 1998;76(9):637–47.

3. Zikusoka MN, Kidd M, Eick G, et al. The molecular genetics of gastroenteropancreatic neuroendocrine tumors. Cancer. 2005;104(11):2292–309.

4. Naswa N, Sharma P, Kumar A, et al. Gallium-68-DOTA-NOC PET/CT of patients with gastroenteropancreatic neuroendocrine tumors: a prospective single-center study. AJR Am J Roentgenol. 2011;197(5):1221–8.

5. Reubi JC. Somatostatin receptors in the gastrointestinal tract in health and disease. Yale J Biol Med. 1992;65(5):493–503; discussion 31-6.

6. Reubi JC. Peptide receptor expression in GEP-NET. Virchows Arch. 2007;451(Suppl 1):S47–50.

7. Williams ED, Sandler M. The classification of carcinoid tumours. Lancet. 1963;1(7275):238–9.

8. Plockinger U, Gustafsson B, Ivan D, et al. ENETS consensus guidelines for the standards of care in neuroendocrine tumors: echocardiography. Neuroendocrinology. 2009;90(2):190–3.

9. Rindi G, Kloppel G, Couvelard A, et al. TNM staging of midgut and hindgut (neuro) endocrine tumors: a consensus proposal including a grading system. Virchows Arch. 2007;451(4):757–62.

10. Rindi G, Kloppel G, Alhman H, et al. TNM staging of foregut (neuro)endocrine tumors: a consensus proposal including a grading system. Virchows Arch. 2006;449(4):395–401.

11. Perren A, Couvelard A, Scoazec JY, et al. ENETS consensus guidelines for the standards of care in neuroendocrine tumors: pathology: diagnosis and prognostic stratification. Neuroendocrinology. 2017;105(3):196–200.

12. Quaedvlieg PF, Visser O, Lamers CB, et al. Epidemiology and survival in patients with carcinoid disease in The Netherlands. An epidemiological study with 2391 patients. Ann Oncol. 2001;12(9):1295–300.

13. Modlin IM, Lye KD, Kidd M. A 5-decade analysis of 13,715 carcinoid tumors. Cancer. 2003;97(4):934–59.

14. Janson ET, Holmberg L, Stridsberg M, et al. Carcinoid tumors: analysis of prognostic factors and survival in 301 patients from a referral center. Ann Oncol. 1997;8(7):685–90.

15. Reubi JC, Waser B, Schaer JC, et al. Somatostatin receptor sst1-sst5 expression in normal and neoplastic human tissues using receptor autoradiography with subtype-selective ligands. Eur J Nucl Med. 2001;28(7):836–46.

16. Behr TM, Gotthardt M, Barth A, et al. Imaging tumors with peptide-based radioligands. Q J Nucl Med. 2001;45(2):189–200.

17. Ambrosini V, Tomassetti P, Franchi R, et al. Imaging of NETs with PET radiopharmaceuticals. Q J Nucl Med Mol Imaging. 2010;54(1):16–23.

18. Bozkurt MF, Virgolini I, Balogova S, et al. Guideline for PET/CT imaging of neuroendocrine neoplasms with (68)Ga-DOTA-conjugated somatostatin receptor targeting peptides and (18)F-DOPA. Eur J Nucl Med Mol Imaging. 2017;44(9):1588–601.

19. Delle Fave G, O'Toole D, Sundin A, et al. ENETS consensus guidelines update for gastroduodenal neuroendocrine neoplasms. Neuroendocrinology. 2016;103(2):119–24.

20. Niederle B, Pape UF, Costa F, et al. ENETS consensus guidelines update for neuroendocrine neoplasms of the jejunum and ileum. Neuroendocrinology. 2016;103(2):125–38.

21. Falconi M, Eriksson B, Kaltsas G, et al. ENETS consensus guidelines update for the management of patients with functional pancreatic neuroendocrine tumors and non-functional pancreatic neuroendocrine tumors. Neuroendocrinology. 2016;103(2):153–71.

22. Garcia-Carbonero R, Sorbye H, Baudin E, et al. ENETS consensus guidelines for high-grade gastroenteropancreatic neuroendocrine tumors and neuroendocrine carcinomas. Neuroendocrinology. 2016;103(2):186–94.

23. Ramage JK, De Herder WW, Delle Fave G, et al. ENETS consensus guidelines update for colorectal neuroendocrine neoplasms. Neuroendocrinology. 2016;103(2):139–43.

24. Pape UF, Niederle B, Costa F, et al. ENETS consensus guidelines for neuroendocrine neoplasms of the appendix (excluding goblet cell carcinomas). Neuroendocrinology. 2016;103(2):144–52.

25. Norton JA, Fraker DL, Alexander HR, et al. Surgery increases survival in patients with gastrinoma. Ann Surg. 2006;244(3):410–9.

26. Akerstrom G. Management of carcinoid tumors of the stomach, duodenum, and pancreas. World J Surg. 1996;20(2):173–82.

27. Rinke A, Muller HH, Schade-Brittinger C, et al. Placebo-controlled, double-blind, prospective, randomized study on the effect of octreotide LAR in the control of tumor growth in patients with metastatic neuroendocrine midgut tumors: a report from the PROMID study group. J Clin Oncol. 2009;27(28):4656–63.

28. Eriksson B, Janson ET, Bax ND, et al. The use of new somatostatin analogues, lanreotide and octastatin, in neuroendocrine gastro-intestinal tumours. Digestion. 1996;57(Suppl 1):77–80.

29. Oberg K, Ferone D, Kaltsas G, et al. ENETS consensus guidelines for the standards of care in neuroendocrine tumors: biotherapy. Neuroendocrinology. 2009;90(2):209–13.

30. Faiss S, Pape UF, Bohmig M, et al. Prospective, randomized, multicenter trial on the antiproliferative effect of lanreotide, interferon alfa, and their combination for therapy of metastatic neuroendocrine gastroenteropancreatic tumors-the International Lanreotide and Interferon Alfa study group. J Clin Oncol. 2003;21(14):2689–96.

31. Eriksson B, Annibale B, Bajetta E, et al. ENETS consensus guidelines for the standards of care in neuroendocrine tumors: chemotherapy in patients with neuroendocrine tumors. Neuroendocrinology. 2009;90(2):214–9.

32. Kouvaraki MA, Ajani JA, Hoff P, et al. Fluorouracil, doxorubicin, and streptozocin in the treatment of patients with locally advanced and metastatic pancreatic endocrine carcinomas. J Clin Oncol. 2004;22(23):4762–71.

33. Pavel ME, Hainsworth JD, Baudin E, et al. Everolimus plus octreotide long-acting repeatable for the treatment of advanced neuroendocrine tumours associated with carcinoid syndrome (RADIANT-2): a randomised, placebo-controlled, phase 3 study. Lancet. 2011;378(9808):2005–12.

34. Yao JC, Phan A, Hoff PM, et al. Targeting vascular endothelial growth factor in advanced carcinoid tumor: a random assignment phase II study of depot octreotide with bevacizumab and pegylated interferon alpha-2b. J Clin Oncol. 2008;26(8):1316–23.

35. Raymond E, Dahan L, Raoul JL, et al. Sunitinib malate for the treatment of pancreatic neuroendocrine tumors. N Engl J Med. 2011;364(6):501–13.

36. Yao JC, Lombard-Bohas C, Baudin E, et al. Daily oral everolimus activity in patients with metastatic pancreatic neuroendocrine tumors after failure of cytotoxic chemotherapy: a phase II trial. J Clin Oncol. 2010;28(1):69–76.

37. Yao JC, Shah MH, Ito T, et al. Everolimus for advanced pancreatic neuroendocrine tumors. N Engl J Med. 2011;364(6):514–23.

38. Patrick DL, Ferketich SL, Frame PS, et al. National institutes of health state-of-the-science conference statement: symptom management in cancer: pain, depression, and fatigue, July 15–17, 2002. J Natl Cancer Inst. 2003;95(15):1110–7.

39. Pavel M, O'Toole D, Costa F, et al. ENETS consensus guidelines update for the management of distant metastatic disease of intestinal, pancreatic, bronchial neuroendocrine neoplasms (NEN) and NEN of unknown primary site. Neuroendocrinology. 2016;103(2):172–85.

40. Krenning EP, de Jong M, Kooij PP, et al. Radiolabelled somatostatin analogue(s) for peptide receptor scintigraphy and radionuclide therapy. Ann Oncol. 1999;10(Suppl 2):S23–9.

41. Bodei L, Handkiewicz-Junak D, Grana C, et al. Receptor radionuclide therapy with 90Y-DOTATOC in patients with medullary thyroid carcinomas. Cancer Biother Radiopharm. 2004;19(1):65–71.

42. Bodei L, Cremonesi M, Grana C, et al. Receptor radionuclide therapy with 90Y-[DOTA]0-Tyr3-octreotide (90Y-DOTATOC) in neuroendocrine tumours. Eur J Nucl Med Mol Imaging. 2004;31(7):1038–46.

43. Valkema R, Pauwels S, Kvols LK, et al. Survival and response after peptide receptor radionuclide therapy with [90Y-DOTA0,Tyr3]octreotide in patients with advanced gastroenteropancreatic neuroendocrine tumors. Semin Nucl Med. 2006;36(2):147–56.

44. Kwekkeboom DJ, Bakker WH, Kam BL, et al. Treatment of patients with gastro-entero-pancreatic (GEP) tumours with the novel radiolabelled somatostatin analogue [177Lu-DOTA(0),Tyr3]octreotate. Eur J Nucl Med Mol Imaging. 2003;30(3):417–22.

45. Waser B, Tamma ML, Cescato R, et al. Highly efficient in vivo agonist-induced internalization of sst2 receptors in somatostatin target tissues. J Nucl Med. 2009;50(6):936–41.

46. Fani M, Nicolas GP, Wild D. Somatostatin receptor antagonists for imaging and therapy. J Nucl Med. 2017;58(Suppl 2):61S–6S.

47. Kwekkeboom D, Krenning EP, de Jong M. Peptide receptor imaging and therapy. J Nucl Med. 2000;41(10):1704–13.

48. Mariani G, Bodei L, Adelstein SJ, et al. Emerging roles for radiometabolic therapy of tumors based on auger electron emission. J Nucl Med. 2000;41(9):1519–21.

49. Janson ET, Westlin JE, Ohrvall U, et al. Nuclear localization of 111In after intravenous injection of [111In-DTPA-D-Phe1]-octreotide in patients with neuroendocrine tumors. J Nucl Med. 2000;41(9):1514–8.

50. Rufini V, Calcagni ML, Baum RP. Imaging of neuroendocrine tumors. Semin Nucl Med. 2006;36(3):228–47.

51. Schottelius M, Wester HJ. Molecular imaging targeting peptide receptors. Methods. 2009; 48(2):161–77.

52. Forrer F, Valkema R, Kwekkeboom DJ, et al. Neuroendocrine tumors. Peptide receptor radionuclide therapy. Best Pract Res Clin Endocrinol Metab. 2007;21(1):111–29.

53. Reubi JC, Schar JC, Waser B, et al. Affinity profiles for human somatostatin receptor subtypes SST1-SST5 of somatostatin radiotracers selected for scintigraphic and radiotherapeutic use. Eur J Nucl Med. 2000;27(3):273–82.

54. Krenning EP, Kwekkeboom DJ, Bakker WH, et al. Somatostatin receptor scintigraphy with [111In-DTPA-D-Phe1]- and [123I-Tyr3]-octreotide: the Rotterdam experience with more than 1000 patients. Eur J Nucl Med. 1993;20(8):716–31.

55. Fjalling M, Andersson P, Forssell-Aronsson E, et al. Systemic radionuclide therapy using indium-111-DTPA-D-Phe1-octreotide in midgut carcinoid syndrome. J Nucl Med. 1996;37(9):1519–21.

56. Valkema R, De Jong M, Bakker WH, et al. Phase I study of peptide receptor radionuclide therapy with [In-DTPA]octreotide: the Rotterdam experience. Semin Nucl Med. 2002;32(2):110–22.

57. Krenning EP, Kooij PP, Bakker WH, et al. Radiotherapy with a radiolabeled somatostatin analogue, [111In-DTPA-D-Phe1]-octreotide. A case history. Ann N Y Acad Sci. 1994;733:496–506.

58. Anthony LB, Woltering EA, Espenan GD, et al. Indium-111-pentetreotide prolongs survival in gastroenteropancreatic malignancies. Semin Nucl Med. 2002;32(2):123–32.

59. Delpassand ES, Sims-Mourtada J, Saso H, et al. Safety and efficacy of radionuclide therapy with high-activity In-111 pentetreotide in patients with progressive neuroendocrine tumors. Cancer Biother Radiopharm. 2008;23(3):292–300.

60. Oberg K, Eriksson B. Endocrine tumours of the pancreas. Best Pract Res Clin Gastroenterol. 2005;19(5):753–81.

61. Mardirossian G, Wu C, Hnatowich DJ. The stability in liver homogenates of indium-111 and yttrium-90 attached to antibody via two popular chelators. Nucl Med Biol. 1993;20(1):65–74.

62. Liu S, Edwards DS. Stabilization of (90)y-labeled DOTA-biomolecule conjugates using gentisic acid and ascorbic acid. Bioconjug Chem. 2001;12(4):554–8.

63. Otte A, Jermann E, Behe M, et al. DOTATOC: a powerful new tool for receptor-mediated radionuclide therapy. Eur J Nucl Med. 1997;24(7):792–5.

64. Otte A, Mueller-Brand J, Dellas S, et al. Yttrium-90-labelled somatostatin-analogue for cancer treatment. Lancet. 1998;351(9100):417–8.

65. Otte A, Herrmann R, Heppeler A, et al. Yttrium-90 DOTATOC: first clinical results. Eur J Nucl Med. 1999;26(11):1439–47.

66. Waldherr C, Pless M, Maecke HR, et al. The clinical value of [90Y-DOTA]-D-Phe1-Tyr3-octreotide (90Y-DOTATOC) in the treatment of neuroendocrine tumours: a clinical phase II study. Ann Oncol. 2001;12(7):941–5.

67. Waldherr C, Pless M, Maecke HR, et al. Tumor response and clinical benefit in neuroendocrine tumors after 7.4 GBq (90)Y-DOTATOC. J Nucl Med. 2002;43(5):610–6.

68. Forrer F, Waldherr C, Maecke HR, et al. Targeted radionuclide therapy with 90Y-DOTATOC in patients with neuroendocrine tumors. Anticancer Res. 2006;26(1B):703–7.

69. Bodei L, Cremonesi M, Zoboli S, et al. Receptor-mediated radionuclide therapy with 90Y-DOTATOC in association with amino acid infusion: a phase I study. Eur J Nucl Med Mol Imaging. 2003;30(2):207–16.

70. De Jong M, Valkema R, Jamar F, et al. Somatostatin receptor-targeted radionuclide therapy of tumors: preclinical and clinical findings. Semin Nucl Med. 2002;32(2):133–40.

71. Virgolini I, Britton K, Buscombe J, et al. In- and Y-DOTA-lanreotide: results and implications of the MAURITIUS trial. Semin Nucl Med. 2002;32(2):148–55.

72. Cwikla JB, Sankowski A, Seklecka N, et al. Efficacy of radionuclide treatment DOTATATE Y-90 in patients with progressive metastatic gastroenteropancreatic neuroendocrine carcinomas (GEP-NETs): a phase II study. Ann Oncol. 2010;21(4):787–94.

73. Kwekkeboom DJ, de Herder WW, Kam BL, et al. Treatment with the radiolabeled somatostatin analog [177 Lu-DOTA 0,Tyr3]octreotate: toxicity, efficacy, and survival. J Clin Oncol. 2008;26(13):2124–30.

74. Strosberg J, El-Haddad G, Wolin E, et al. Phase 3 trial of (177)Lu-Dotatate for midgut neuroendocrine tumors. N Engl J Med. 2017;376(2):125–35.

75. Strosberg J, Wolin E, Chasen B, et al. Health-related quality of life in patients with progressive midgut neuroendocrine tumors treated with (177) Lu-Dotatate in the phase III NETTER-1 trial. J Clin Oncol. 2018;36(25):2578–84.

76. de Jong M, Breeman WA, Valkema R, et al. Combination radionuclide therapy using 177Lu- and 90Y-labeled somatostatin analogs. J Nucl Med. 2005;46(Suppl 1):13S–7S.

77. Villard L, Romer A, Marincek N, et al. Cohort study of somatostatin-based radiopeptide therapy with [(90)Y-DOTA]-TOC versus [(90)Y-DOTA]-TOC plus [(177)Lu-DOTA]-TOC in neuroendocrine cancers. J Clin Oncol. 2012;30(10):1100–6.

78. Kunikowska J, Krolicki L, Hubalewska-Dydejczyk A, et al. Clinical results of radionuclide therapy of neuroendocrine tumours with 90Y-DOTATATE and tandem 90Y/177Lu-DOTATATE: which is a better therapy option? Eur J Nucl Med Mol Imaging. 2011;38(10):1788–97.

79. Pool SE, Kam BL, Koning GA, et al. [(111) In-DTPA]octreotide tumor uptake in GEPNET liver metastases after intra-arterial administration: an overview of preclinical and clinical observations and implications for tumor radiation dose after peptide radionuclide therapy. Cancer Biother Radiopharm. 2014;29(4):179–87.

80. Hofman MS, Hicks RJ. Peptide receptor radionuclide therapy for neuroendocrine tumours: standardized and randomized, or personalized? Eur J Nucl Med Mol Imaging. 2014;41(2):211–3.

81. van Essen M, Krenning EP, Kam BL, et al. Report on short-term side effects of treatments with 177Lu-octreotate in combination with capecitabine in seven patients with gastroenteropancreatic neuroendocrine tumours. Eur J Nucl Med Mol Imaging. 2008;35(4):743–8.

82. Hubble D, Kong G, Michael M, et al. 177Lu-octreotate, alone or with radiosensitising chemotherapy, is safe in neuroendocrine tumour patients previously treated with high-activity 111In-octreotide. Eur J Nucl Med Mol Imaging. 2010;37(10):1869–75.

83. Claringbold PG, Brayshaw PA, Price RA, et al. Phase II study of radiopeptide 177Lu-octreotate and capecitabine therapy of progressive disseminated neuroendocrine tumours. Eur J Nucl Med Mol Imaging. 2011;38(2):302–11.

84. Kashyap R, Hofman MS, Michael M, et al. Favourable outcomes of (177)Lu-octreotate peptide receptor chemoradionuclide therapy in patients with FDG-avid neuroendocrine tumours. Eur J Nucl Med Mol Imaging. 2015;42(2):176–85.

85. Claringbold PG, Price RA, Turner JH. Phase I-II study of radiopeptide 177Lu-octreotate in combination with capecitabine and temozolomide in advanced low-grade neuroendocrine tumors. Cancer Biother Radiopharm. 2012;27(9):561–9.

86. Rashidi A, Sorscher SM. Temozolomide-associated myelodysplasia 6 years after treatment of a patient with pancreatic neuroendocrine tumor. Leuk Lymphoma. 2015;56(8):2468–9.

87. Forrer F, Uusijarvi H, Storch D, et al. Treatment with 177Lu-DOTATOC of patients with relapse of neuroendocrine tumors after treatment with 90Y-DOTATOC. J Nucl Med. 2005;46(8):1310–6.

88. Frilling A, Weber F, Saner F, et al. Treatment with (90)Y- and (177)Lu-DOTATOC in patients with metastatic neuroendocrine tumors. Surgery. 2006;140(6):968–76; discussion 76–7.

89. Severi S, Sansovini M, Ianniello A, et al. Feasibility and utility of re-treatment with (177)Lu-DOTATATE in GEP-NENs relapsed after treatment with (90)Y-DOTATOC. Eur J Nucl Med Mol Imaging. 2015;42(13):1955–63.

90. Brans B, Bodei L, Giammarile F, et al. Clinical radionuclide therapy dosimetry: the quest for the "Holy Gray". Eur J Nucl Med Mol Imaging. 2007;34(5):772–86.

91. Stabin MG, Sparks RB, Crowe E. OLINDA/EXM: the second-generation personal computer software for internal dose assessment in nuclear medicine. J Nucl Med. 2005;46(6):1023–7.

92. Pauwels S, Barone R, Walrand S, et al. Practical dosimetry of peptide receptor radionuclide therapy with (90)Y-labeled somatostatin analogs. J Nucl Med. 2005;46(Suppl 1):92S–8S.

93. Jamar F, Barone R, Mathieu I, et al. (86Y-DOTA0)-D-Phe1-Tyr3-octreotide (SMT487)-a phase 1 clinical study: pharmacokinetics, biodistribution and renal protective effect of different regimens of amino acid co-infusion. Eur J Nucl Med Mol Imaging. 2003;30(4):510–8.

94. Barone R, Borson-Chazot F, Valkema R, et al. Patient-specific dosimetry in predicting renal toxicity with (90)Y-DOTATOC: relevance of kidney volume and dose rate in finding a dose-effect relationship. J Nucl Med. 2005;46(Suppl 1):99S–106S.

95. DeNardo GL, Juweid ME, White CA, et al. Role of radiation dosimetry in radioimmunotherapy planning and treatment dosing. Crit Rev Oncol Hematol. 2001;39(1–2):203–18.

96. Cremonesi M, Botta F, Di Dia A, et al. Dosimetry for treatment with radiolabelled somatostatin analogues. A review. Q J Nucl Med Mol Imaging. 2010;54(1):37–51.

97. Forrer F, Uusijarvi H, Waldherr C, et al. A comparison of (111)In-DOTATOC and (111)In-DOTATATE: biodistribution and dosimetry in the same patients with metastatic neuroendocrine tumours. Eur J Nucl Med Mol Imaging. 2004;31(9):1257–62.

98. Fabbri C, Sarti G, Cremonesi M, et al. Quantitative analysis of 90Y Bremsstrahlung SPECT-CT images for application to 3D patient-specific dosimetry. Cancer Biother Radiopharm. 2009;24(1):145–54.

99. Lhommel R, Goffette P, Van den Eynde M, et al. Yttrium-90 TOF PET scan demonstrates high-resolution biodistribution after liver SIRT. Eur J Nucl Med Mol Imaging. 2009;36(10):1696.

100. Forrer F, Krenning EP, Kooij PP, et al. Bone marrow dosimetry in peptide receptor radionuclide therapy with [177Lu-DOTA(0),Tyr(3)]octreotate. Eur J Nucl Med Mol Imaging. 2009;36(7):1138–46.

101. Konijnenberg M, Melis M, Valkema R, et al. Radiation dose distribution in human kidneys by octreotides in peptide receptor radionuclide therapy. J Nucl Med. 2007;48(1):134–42.

102. Forrer F, Rolleman E, Bijster M, et al. From outside to inside? Dose-dependent renal tubular damage after high-dose peptide receptor radionuclide therapy in rats measured with in vivo (99m)Tc-DMSA-SPECT and molecular imaging. Cancer Biother Radiopharm. 2007;22(1):40–9.

103. de Jong M, Barone R, Krenning E, et al. Megalin is essential for renal proximal tubule reabsorption of (111)In-DTPA-octreotide. J Nucl Med. 2005;46(10):1696–700.

104. De Jong M, Valkema R, Van Gameren A, et al. Inhomogeneous localization of radioactivity in the human kidney after injection of [(111)In-DTPA] octreotide. J Nucl Med. 2004;45(7):1168–71.

105. Konijnenberg MW, Bijster M, Krenning EP, et al. A stylized computational model of the rat for organ dosimetry in support of preclinical evaluations of peptide receptor radionuclide therapy with (90)Y, (111)In, or (177)Lu. J Nucl Med. 2004;45(7):1260–9.

106. Bodei L, Cremonesi M, Ferrari M, et al. Long-term evaluation of renal toxicity after peptide receptor radionuclide therapy with 90Y-DOTATOC and 177Lu-DOTATATE: the role of associated risk factors. Eur J Nucl Med Mol Imaging. 2008;35(10):1847–56.

107. Valkema R, Pauwels SA, Kvols LK, et al. Long-term follow-up of renal function after peptide receptor radiation therapy with (90)Y-DOTA(0),Tyr(3)-octreotide and (177)Lu-DOTA(0), Tyr(3)-octreotate. J Nucl Med. 2005;46(Suppl 1):83S–91S.

108. Hicks RJ, Kwekkeboom DJ, Krenning E, et al. ENETS consensus guidelines for the standards of care in neuroendocrine neoplasia: peptide receptor radionuclide therapy with radiolabeled somatostatin analogues. Neuroendocrinology. 2017;105(3):295–309.

109. Bodei L, Mueller-Brand J, Baum RP, et al. The joint IAEA, EANM, and SNMMI practical guidance on peptide receptor radionuclide therapy (PRRNT) in neuroendocrine tumours. Eur J Nucl Med Mol Imaging. 2013;40(5):800–16.

110. Barone R, Pauwels S, De Camps J, et al. Metabolic effects of amino acid solutions infused for renal protection during therapy with radiolabelled somatostatin analogues. Nephrol Dial Transplant. 2004;19(9):2275–81.

111. Rolleman EJ, Valkema R, de Jong M, et al. Safe and effective inhibition of renal uptake of radiolabelled octreotide by a combination of lysine and arginine. Eur J Nucl Med Mol Imaging. 2003;30(1):9–15.

112. Giovacchini G, Nicolas G, Freidank H, et al. Effect of amino acid infusion on potassium serum levels in neuroendocrine tumour patients treated with

targeted radiopeptide therapy. Eur J Nucl Med Mol Imaging. 2011;38(9):1675–82.

113. Bernard BF, Krenning EP, Breeman WA, et al. D-lysine reduction of indium-111 octreotide and yttrium-90 octreotide renal uptake. J Nucl Med. 1997;38(12):1929–33.

114. Rolleman EJ, Melis M, Valkema R, et al. Kidney protection during peptide receptor radionuclide therapy with somatostatin analogues. Eur J Nucl Med Mol Imaging. 2010;37(5):1018–31.

115. Rolleman EJ, Forrer F, Bernard B, et al. Amifostine protects rat kidneys during peptide receptor radionuclide therapy with [177Lu-DOTA0,Tyr3]octreotate. Eur J Nucl Med Mol Imaging. 2007;34(5):763–71.

116. Imhof A, Brunner P, Marincek N, et al. Response, survival, and long-term toxicity after therapy with the radiolabeled somatostatin analogue [90Y-DOTA]-TOC in metastasized neuroendocrine cancers. J Clin Oncol. 2011;29(17):2416–23.

117. Sabet A, Ezziddin K, Pape UF, et al. Long-term hematotoxicity after peptide receptor radionuclide therapy with 177Lu-octreotate. J Nucl Med. 2013;54(11):1857–61.

118. Brieau B, Hentic O, Lebtahi R, et al. High risk of myelodysplastic syndrome and acute myeloid leukemia after 177Lu-octreotate PRRT in NET patients heavily pretreated with alkylating chemotherapy. Endocr Relat Cancer. 2016;23(5):L17–23.

119. Sierra ML, Agazzi A, Bodei L, et al. Lymphocytic toxicity in patients after peptide-receptor radionuclide therapy (PRRT) with 177Lu-DOTATATE and 90Y-DOTATOC. Cancer Biother Radiopharm. 2009;24(6):659–65.

120. Esser JP, Krenning EP, Teunissen JJ, et al. Comparison of [(177)Lu-DOTA(0),Tyr(3)]octreotate and [(177)Lu-DOTA(0),Tyr(3)]octreotide: which peptide is preferable for PRRT? Eur J Nucl Med Mol Imaging. 2006;33(11):1346–51.

121. Benua RS, Cicale NR, Sonenberg M, et al. The relation of radioiodine dosimetry to results and complications in the treatment of metastatic thyroid cancer. Am J Roentgenol Radium Therapy, Nucl Med. 1962;87:171–82.

122. Cremonesi M, Ferrari M, Bodei L, et al. Dosimetry in peptide radionuclide receptor therapy: a review. J Nucl Med. 2006;47(9):1467–75.

123. Bushnell D, Menda Y, Madsen M, et al. Assessment of hepatic toxicity from treatment with 90Y-SMT 487 (OctreoTher(TM)) in patients with diffuse somatostatin receptor positive liver metastases. Cancer Biother Radiopharm. 2003;18(4):581–8.

124. Kwekkeboom DJ, Mueller-Brand J, Paganelli G, et al. Overview of results of peptide receptor radionuclide therapy with 3 radiolabeled somatostatin analogs. J Nucl Med. 2005;46(Suppl 1):62S–6S.

125. Riff BP, Yang YX, Soulen MC, et al. Peptide receptor radionuclide therapy-induced hepatotoxicity in patients with metastatic neuroendocrine tumors. Clin Nucl Med. 2015;40(11):845–50.

126. Teunissen JJ, Krenning EP, de Jong FH, et al. Effects of therapy with [177Lu-DOTA 0,Tyr 3]octreotate on endocrine function. Eur J Nucl Med Mol Imaging. 2009;36(11):1758–66.

127. Brunner P, Jorg AC, Glatz K, et al. The prognostic and predictive value of sstr2-immunohistochemistry and sstr2-targeted imaging in neuroendocrine tumors. Eur J Nucl Med Mol Imaging. 2017;44(3):468–75.

128. Kwekkeboom DJ, Teunissen JJ, Bakker WH, et al. Radiolabeled somatostatin analog [177Lu-DOTA0,Tyr3]octreotate in patients with endocrine gastroenteropancreatic tumors. J Clin Oncol. 2005;23(12):2754–62.

129. Clancy TE, Sengupta TP, Paulus J, et al. Alkaline phosphatase predicts survival in patients with metastatic neuroendocrine tumors. Dig Dis Sci. 2006;51(5):877–84.

130. Binderup T, Knigge U, Loft A, et al. 18F-fluorodeoxyglucose positron emission tomography predicts survival of patients with neuroendocrine tumors. Clin Cancer Res. 2010; 16(3):978–85.

131. Garin E, Le Jeune F, Devillers A, et al. Predictive value of 18F-FDG PET and somatostatin receptor scintigraphy in patients with metastatic endocrine tumors. J Nucl Med. 2009;50(6):858–64.

^{131}I-MIBG Therapy of Malignant Neuroblastoma and Pheochromocytoma

5

Arnoldo Piccardo, Luca Foppiani, Sergio Righi, Alberto Garaventa, Stefania Sorrentino, and Egesta Lopci

5.1 Neuroblastoma

5.1.1 Basis

Neuroblastoma (NB) represents the most frequent extracranial tumor of pediatric age. It derives from aberrant neural crest development and presents as an abdominal, thoracic, or neck masses originating in the adrenal medulla or paraspinal sympathetic ganglia [1]. A primary tumor is not found in approximately 1% of patients, in whom the disease becomes apparent only through signs of metastatic spread. Peripheral neuroblastic tumors is the correct term to identify the group of neural crest-derived

A. Piccardo (✉)
Department of Nuclear Medicine and PET/CT Centre, Oncology Institute of Southern Switzerland, Bellinzona, Switzerland

Department of Nuclear Medicine, E.O. Ospedali Galliera, Genoa, Italy
e-mail: arnoldo.piccardo@galliera.it

L. Foppiani
Internal Medicine, Galliera Hospital, Genoa, Italy

S. Righi
Medical Physics Department, E.O. Galliera Hospital, Genoa, Italy

A. Garaventa · S. Sorrentino
Unit of Pediatric Oncology, Gaslini Hospital, Genoa, Italy

E. Lopci
Department of Nuclear Medicine, Humanitas Research Hospital, Milan, Italy

embryonal tumors including neuroblastoma, ganglioneuroblastoma, and ganglioneuroma [2]. Peripheral neuroblastic tumors represent 6–10% of all pediatric cancers (age 0–14 yrs). The age distribution is characterized by a peak of incidence in the first year of life (infants), followed by a rapid decline in the following years. After the age of 6, it becomes rare and exceptional among adolescents and adults. NB occurs at slightly higher rates in males than in females (M/F ratio 1.1–1.2) and its mean annual incidence is 7–12 cases per million children in Western countries [3].

More than 90% of NB excrete catecholamines, which, together with their metabolites, are used for diagnostic and follow-up purposes [2].

A familial history of neuroblastoma is observed in approximately 1% of patients with an estimated penetrance of 11% in hereditary cases. Two main neural crest-derived developmental disorders are associated with an increased risk to develop neuroblastoma: (1) Hirschsprung's disease, characterized by an absence of ganglion cells in the distal colon resulting in functional obstruction and (2) Ondine's curse, also named congenital central hypoventilation syndrome, a disorder characterized by a failure of the autonomic control of ventilation during sleep. Both diseases are frequently associated with each other, and most cases are linked to mutation of the *PHOX2B* gene [4].

Recently, the anaplastic lymphoma kinase (*ALK*) gene was identified as a second neuroblastoma predisposition gene. ALK mutations are present in around 9% of primary NB tumors and approximately 14% of high-risk setting [5].

Although neuroblastomas may occur in familial and syndromic contexts, most cases occur sporadically. However, also in this context, the amplification of oncogenes, as MYCN, is clinically relevant because it is associated with advanced stage disease and rapid tumor progression, and the *MYCN* oncogene status is routinely used in clinical practice to assign therapeutic intensity.

The clinical presentation of NB is heterogeneous, ranging from asymptomatic incidental tumors to spontaneously regressing metastatic tumors in infancy or to widespread metastatic disease progressing to death despite intensive therapy. At diagnosis, patients with metastatic neuroblastic tumors usually present constitutional symptoms such as pain, fever, and decay of the overall health status. The main metastatic sites are regional lymph nodes, bone, and bone marrow.

Due to the heterogeneous profile of the disease, prognosis of NB patients is linked to several clinical and biological factors. In this setting the International Neuroblastoma Risk Group (INRG) task force established criteria for an internationally risk group stratification system based on clinical factors as age, tumor stage (Table 5.1 and 5.2), and genetic determinants (MYCN gene amplification, chromosome 1p36 abnormalities) (Table 5.3) [1, 6].

Table 5.1 International neuroblastoma staging system (INSS) [19]

NB	Tumor	Resection	Lymph node
Stage 1	Localized	Complete	Ipsilateral and negative
Stage 2A	Localized	Incomplete	Ipsilateral and negative
Stage 2B	Localized	Complete or incomplete	Ipsilateral and positive
Stage 3	Localized across the midline	Unresectable	With or without involvement
Stage 4	Any	Any	Distant metastases

Table 5.2 International neuroblastoma risk group (INRG) staging system [1]

Stage	Description
L1	Localized tumor not involving vital structures and confined to one body compartment
L2	Loco-regional tumor with presence of one or more image-defined risk-factors
M	Distant metastatic disease (except stage MS)
MS	Metastatic disease in children younger than 18 months with metastases confined to skin, liver, and/or bone marrow

More recently, the INRG Task Force also released the consensus recommendations on molecular techniques, on the criteria of minimal residual disease, on neuroblastoma response criteria, and on radiographic techniques [6–10].

The high-risk phenotype, which affects nearly 50% of newly diagnosed patients and is related to poor long-term survival, is characterized by age >18 months on diagnosis, widespread disease dissemination, and MYCN amplification. Conversely, patients with a low-risk phenotype (no MYCN amplification and age <18 months) have an excellent long-term survival [11–13].

Localized unresectable neuroblastoma in children >12 months and no MYCN amplification constitute an intermediate risk group [14].

Since risk group stratification is an essential step to select the most appropriate treatment option, diagnostic imaging is determinant in the initial assessment of disease extension.

In this setting, nuclear medicine procedures, by using meta-iodobenzylguanidine (mIBG) imaging, have been reported to be very effective especially in evaluating bone and bone marrow NB involvement at the time of diagnosis and during treatment [15].

mIBG is a noradrenaline analogue developed in the late 1970s as diagnostic agent for imaging of adrenal medulla [16]. MIBG is chemically related to norepinephrine and its uptake in the cytoplasm of NB cells is associated to the amine type-1 uptake mechanism. Indeed, mIBG and norepinephrine share similar specific active uptake mechanism [17].

^{123}I-mIBG scintigraphy and ^{131}I-mIBG scintigraphy have been extensively used in research

Table 5.3 International neuroblastoma risk groups consensus pretreatment classification schema [6]

INRG stage	Age (months)	Histological classification	Grade of tumor differentiation	MYCN	11q Aberration	Ploidy	Pretreatment risk group
L1/ L2	Any	GN maturing GNB intermixed					Very Low
L1	Any	Any except GN maturing or GNB intermixed		NA			Very Low
				Amp			High
L2	<18	Any except GN maturing or GNB intermixed		NA	No		Low
					Yes		Intermediate
	≥18	GNB nodular; neuroblastoma	Differentiating	NA	No		Low
			Poorly differentiating or undifferentiating	NA	Yes		Intermediate
M	< 18			NA		Hyperdiploid	Low
	<12			NA		Diploid	Intermediate
	12 to <18			NA		Diploid	Intermediate
	< 18			Amp			High
	≥ 18						High
MS	< 18			NA	No		Very Low
					Yes		High
				Amp			High

GN ganglioneuroma, *GNB* ganglioneuroblastoma, *Amp* amplified, *NA* not amplified

and clinical imaging of NB and are both well-established diagnostic methods in the diagnosis, staging, and restaging of NB. Indeed, ^{123}I-MIBG scintigraphy has been recognized as the functional imaging of choice in NB assessment and has been widely used in clinical practice for the past 25 years.

Owing to the high specificity and sensitivity in detecting primary NB and distant metastases, mIBG imaging is recommended as standard modality to assess disease extent at diagnosis and to identify the risk of the each patient according to International Neuroblastoma Risk Group (INRG) guidance [18].

Worthy to remember, in INRG recommendations the presence of a single, unequivocal mIBG-positive lesion at a distant site is sufficient to define metastatic disease [5]. Consequently, since 1996 mIBG scan has been utilized to create a risk-factor scoring system focusing on the extent and treatment response of bone disease [19–23].

Moreover, the presence of a positive ^{123}I-mIBG scan establishes the basis for the use of a targeted radionuclide therapy with ^{131}I-mIBG.

5.1.2 Therapeutic Context, Indication, and Results of ^{131}I-mIBG Therapy

The majority (>80%) of patients with high-risk NB are >18 months of age with INRG stage M disease, as well as children 12–18 months of age with INRG stage M disease, whose tumors have unfavorable biological features (MYCN amplification, unfavorable pathology and/or diploid) [24]. The current approach for high-risk NB incorporates induction chemotherapy (to reduce tumor burden by shrinking the primary tumor and reducing metastases) using a combination chemotherapy regimen, followed by delayed surgery to remove the primary tumor and subsequent myeloablative chemotherapy associated to autologous hematopoietic stem cell transplantation (AHSCT) [24]. Myeloablative chemotherapy is followed by maintenance therapy for minimal residual disease with anti-GD2 monoclonal antibody and cytokine immune therapy, in addition to differentiating therapy with isotretinoin (Fig. 5.1) [24].

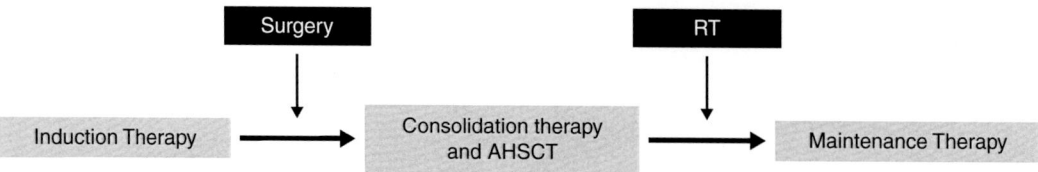

Fig. 5.1 Treatment of high-risk neuroblastoma. Induction therapy includes combination chemotherapy) and a peripheral blood stem cell harvest. Surgery approach is attempted after chemotherapy. A high-dose chemotherapy with autologous hematopoietic stem cell transplantation (AHSCT) is useful to eliminate remaining disease. Radiotherapy to the primary tumor bed and maintenance therapy for minimal residual disease by using anti-GD2 antibody and isotretinoin are introduced at the end of the therapeutic *iter* [24]

Although some studies evaluated the role of mIBG therapeutic approach at the time of the first induction [25, 26] or at the time of consolidation [27], the main indication for ^{131}I-mIBG therapy is in high-risk NB patients with evidence of persistence of mIBG avid metastatic disease at the end of the long therapeutic "iter" described above (Fig. 5.2).

No strict inclusion or exclusion criteria are reported in literature but an adequate life expectancy of at least 3 months and a preserved renal function should be required. In addition, hematopoietic parameters (WBC > 3000/μL, Platelets >100 K/μL) should also be considered before ^{131}I-mIBG therapy, especially when stem cells are not available [28]. In the presence of normal renal function there is no limitation in treating previously nephrectomized patients for large adrenal masses.

No prospective, randomized and controlled trials have been conducted to identify the correct indication for mIBG therapy. Indeed, at least 27 studies, treating 911 relapsing or refractory NB patients with ^{131}I-mIBG, have been analyzed in a recent systematic review by Wilson and colleagues [29]. They found that the overall mean tumor response rate was 32% although a wide range of proportions for each study has been reported [29]. In this context, tumor response was 39% in patients who had also concomitant chemotherapy compared to 32% for those patients treated with ^{131}I-mIBG alone. No difference was observed when refractory and relapse patients were compared (response rate 37% vs. 38%) (Figs. 5.3 and 5.4). When was considered the cumulative activity of ^{131}I-mIBG and the association between chemotherapy and mIBG both parameters were found positively associated to treatment response [28].

The median overall survival reported only in seven [30–36] of the 27 studies ranged from 6 months to 48 months. Among these 27 studies only four had controls arms [31, 33, 37, 38]. Survival outcomes were similar between patients treated with mIBG therapy and controls in three of these four studies, with median survival around 6 months. On the other hand, Miano and colleagues reported that patients treated with ^{131}I-mIBG had a longer event-free survival (EFS) (18 vs. 3 months) [37].

The largest mIBG therapy study conducted on 164 refractory or relapsed NB patients in 2007 by Matthay and colleagues, by using an activity of 12–18 mCi/Kg, showed that the overall response rate (including only complete and partial response) was 36% [32]. Indeed, the response rate for the 12-mCi/Kg cohort was 25%, and the 18-mCi/Kg cohort was 37%.

They found, at multivariate level, that the principal parameters influencing the response to treatment, were age (patients with more than 6 years had a significantly higher likelihood of response and longer EFS than younger patients), disease limited to either soft tissue or to bone and bone marrow only, and less prior treatment (less than 3 previous regimens). In addition, the authors found that a longer time from diagnosis to mIBG therapy, often related to a less aggressive disease, is another parameter positively associated to treatment response.

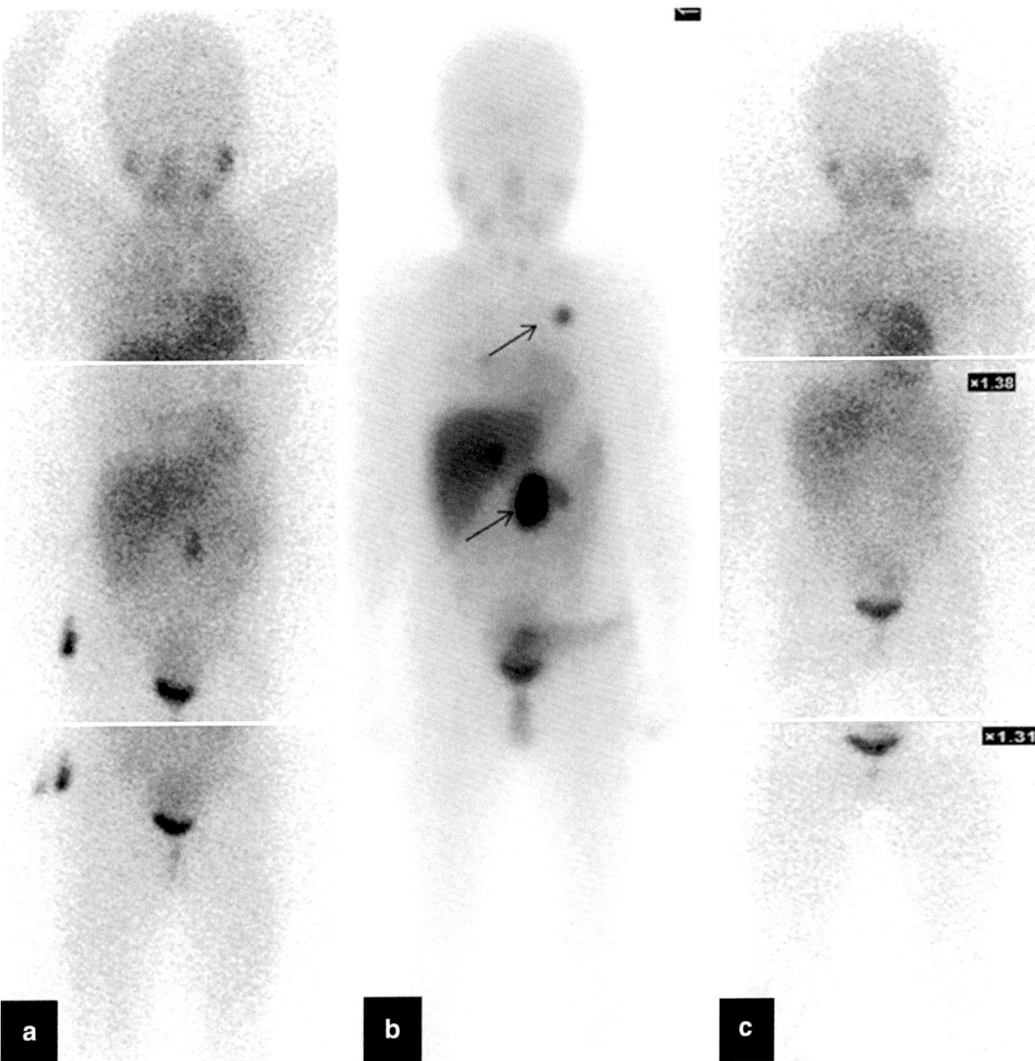

Fig. 5.2 Five years old male affected by stage IV NB. Patient showed persistence of disease after NB AR 01 protocol on ^{123}I-mIBG whole body scintigraphy (**a**). Patients underwent ^{131}I mIBG therapy (15 mCi/Kg) and post-therapeutic whole body scintigraphy (**b**) confirmed one metastasis of the left lung and the unresectable primary tumor (arrows). Three months later, ^{123}I-mIBG whole-body scintigraphy (**c**) demonstrated optimal metabolic response to treatment

5.1.3 Risk and Complications of the Procedure, Side Effects

^{131}I-mIBG infusion is a safe therapeutic administration and few peri-procedural complications have been reported. However, some precautions should be considered before administering mIBG therapy. First an adequate hydration of the patient and a proper premedication with antiemetic drugs should be performed. These simple precautions may at the same time increase the urinary excretion of the tracer (i.e., reduction of bladder radiation exposure) and improve the tolerability to mIBG induced actinic gastritis. In order to limit the early ^{131}I-mIBG loss due to deiodination, ^{131}I-mIBG infusion should be fast, not more than an hour, even in the event of

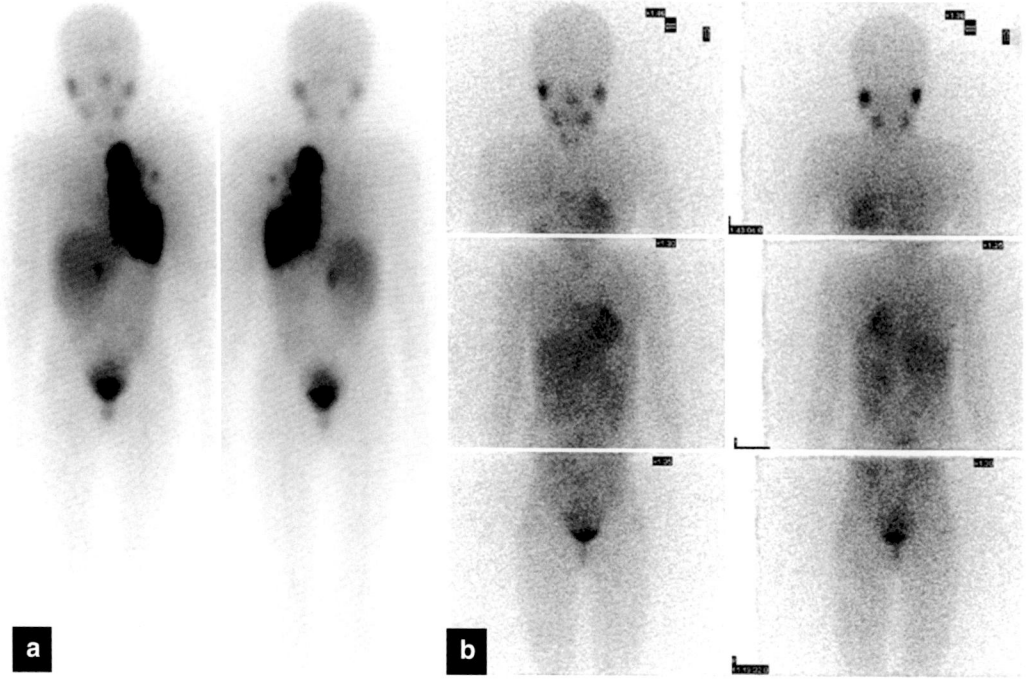

Fig. 5.3 Seven years old female affected by stage IV NB. Patient, after NB AR 01 protocol, showed persistence of disease involving the left lung and pleura. Patient underwent [131]I mIBG therapy (300 mCi) and post-therapeutic whole body scintigraphy (**a**) confirmed the sites of disease. Three months later, ^{123}I-mIBG whole body scintigraphy (**b**) demonstrated optimal metabolic response to treatment

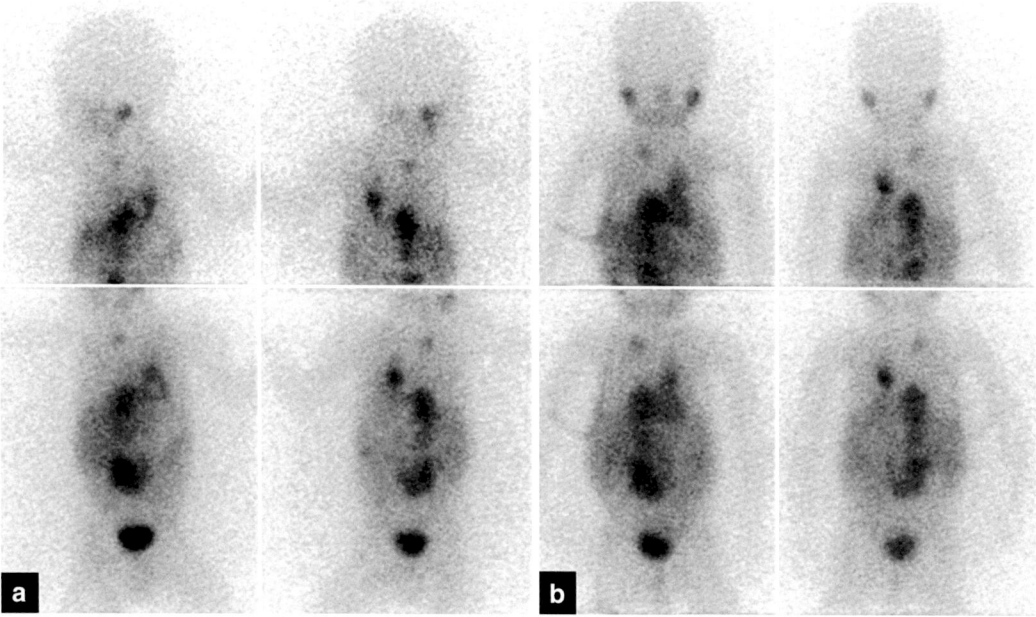

Fig. 5.4 Three years old male affected by stage IV NB. Patient, after NB AR 01 protocol, showed persistence of disease on ^{123}I-mIBG whole body scintigraphy (**a**). Patient underwent [131]I mIBG therapy (15 mCi/Kg) but 3 months later a diagnostic ^{123}I-mIBG whole body scintigraphy (**b**) did not show any significant response to treatment

Table 5.4 Principal side effects and toxicities in NB patients treated with mIBG therapy

Impact	Acute	Early	Late
Frequent	Nausea	Thrombocytopenia	Hypothyroidism
Less Frequent	Anorexia	Leukopenia	Papillary Thyroid Cancer
Infrequent	Vomiting	Neutropenia	Other second malignancies

very high activities injected [39]. Close 131I-mIBG cycles have been proposed and the principal limitation of this approach is related to the total amount of activity administered. However, repeated treatments are well tolerated and stunning effect reducing the mIBG uptake has never been reported.

Acute toxicity, occurring within the first hours after the infusion, consists of nausea, anorexia, and vomiting. Transient tachycardia and hypertension are rare and reported in less than 10% of the patients [40] (Table 5.4).

Early hematological toxicity is the major issue but often the entity is not severe and is activity/weight related. Usually it appears 2–4 weeks after infusion but the nadir occurs 2–3 weeks later and the spontaneous recovery can be very slow after 4–6 weeks. As reported by Matthay and colleagues an activity higher than 444 MBq/Kg may be considered, the limit behind which significant hematological events may occur [41]. From this point of view, in these cases, a stem cell support is required.

Among hematological toxicities, the most frequent and severe is persistent thrombocytopenia [30, 42]. However in a recent paper by Bleeker and colleagues was pointed out that grade IV thrombocytopenia occurs in only 1% of patients and no episodes of major bleeding has been observed [43].

Some studies have found a correlation between bone-bone marrow involvement and hematological toxicity. This finding was more recently confirmed by Bleeker [43] reporting that the patients with more severe toxicity (grade IV anemia, leukocytopenia, or thrombocytopenia) all had disseminated bone marrow disease.

Although the thyroid block is a corner stone in the preparation of patients for mIBG therapy, hypothyroidism is a major late side effect, despite the recent introduction of intense of protocol using the combination potassium iodide, methimazole, and L-thyroxine [44]. One recent paper by Clement and colleagues reported at a median follow-up of 9.0 years after 131I-mIBG treatment the presence of thyroid disorders in 50% patients and TSH elevation in 37% [45]. Papillary thyroid cancers may occur with a rather high frequency and in the same recent paper one out of the 24 NB patients survived developed a papillary thyroid cancer [45].

Apart from thyroid cancers, second malignancies are rare and arise in less than 5% [46]. Garaventa and colleagues reported two cases of leukemia, one angiomatoid fibrous histiocytoma, one schwannoma, and one rhabdomyosarcoma in 119 NB patients after 131I-mIBG therapy [47]. Nevertheless, in children heavily treated with a chemotherapy multimodality therapy, it is difficult to distinguish the risk of developing secondary malignancies derived from 131I-mIBG radiation effects and the risk derived from the alkylator-based chemotherapies [40].

5.2 Pheocromocytoma

5.2.1 Basis

Pheochromocytomas (PCCs) and paragangliomas (PPGs) are rare neuroendocrine tumors originating in the adrenal medulla and in the extra-adrenal ganglia, respectively. Their prevalence ranges from 1:2500 to 1:6500 in Western countries, and occur in less than 1% of hypertensive patients [48, 49].

The vast majority of PCCs are benign and malignancy occurs in ~10% of patients; by contrast 20–40% of PPGs are malignant. These tumors are considered malignant only when metastasis is present, since there are no reliable histological features or molecular markers able to differentiate a benign from a malignant tumor. Metastases occur most frequently in lymph nodes (70–80%), bone (50–70%), liver (50%), and lungs (30–50%) and can appear up to 20 years after initial presentation [50, 51]. Notably, patients presenting with only bone metastasis have longer overall survival compared with those with liver and/or lung metastases [52].

The most important molecular predictor of malignancy is the presence of inactivating germline mutations of the mitochondrial succinate dehydrogenase subunit B (SDHB). This mutations result in a hypermethylation phenotype with abnormal activation of epithelial-to-mesenchymal transition, and a more aggressive phenotype [52]. Besides the genotype of the primary tumor (i.e., carrier of SDHB mutations), other factors such as the size and the location (adrenal or extra-adrenal) predict the onset of metastases and overall survival. In particular, PCCs larger than 5 cm and PPGs are at high risk to develop metastases [51].

The natural history of malignant PCCS and PGGs is heterogeneous. In fact, several patients have indolent disease irrespective of the presence of distant metastases, which remain stable over time; these patients may survive for several years with good quality of life and minimal or no therapeutic intervention. On the other hand, some patients show very aggressive disease with huge metastases, no response to systemic therapy, and hence short life expectancy. However, most patients exhibit intermediate outcomes with progressive disease that will require medical/surgical management over time [52]. Overall, patients with metastatic PCC/PGL have a 50% 5-year overall survival [48].

These tumors, mostly PCCs, are frequently characterized by an excessive and often paroxystic secretion of catecholamines which cause symptoms such as palpitations, throbbing headaches, and sweating. Although typical when present, this clinical triad is uncommonly encountered in most patients. In addition, since these symptoms are not specific, the diagnosis of these tumors is frequently overlooked. By contrast, hypertension, particularly if resistant or paroxysmal, must alert the clinicians to the possibility of a pheochromocytoma. In addition, severe hypertension or hypertensive crises following procedures as anesthesia, surgery, or angiography should raise the suspicion of PCC. However up to 10% of patients are normotensive [48, 49].

Finally, orthostatic hypotension due to catecholamine-induced intravascular volume depletion can be an uncommon presenting feature of these tumors. No significant clinical difference occurs between benign and malignant disease.

Up to 60% of malignant PCCs and PPGs patients have tumor burden- and hormone-related manifestations (e.g., pain and hypertension); most of these tumors produce noradrenaline and/or dopamine [51].

Three types of complications significantly affect clinical outcomes and therapeutic choices in metastatic PCCs and PPGs patients: cardiovascular disease, gastrointestinal dysfunction (severe constipation, obstruction, ulceration, perforation, and/or bacterial translocation), and skeletal-related events (SREs) [52]. SREs include pain, pathological fractures, and/or cord compression; although metastases are usually lytic these patients rarely develop hypercalcemia.

With regard to cardiovascular disease, patients with catecholamine secreting tumors are at risk of congestive heart failure, stroke, arrhythmias, and cardiomyopathy.

In addition, chemotherapy, molecular targeted therapies, and radiopharmaceutical agents used to treat these tumors destroy tumoral cells, thus predisposing patients to hypertensive crisis. Consequently, these patients require proper α- and β-adrenergic blockade. Not-competitive α1-adrenergic blockers such as doxazosin and terazosin are commonly used. β-Adrenergic agents (e.g., propranolol, atenolol) should be instituted after the α-adrenergic blockade has been optimized. For bone metastases, a combined approach including analgesics, antiresorptive agents (bisphosphonates or RANK ligand antagonists), steroids, surgery, or radiotherapy is recommended [51].

In malignant PCCs and PGGs surgical resection of the primary tumor, albeit not curative, can have a positive impact on clinical outcomes since it causes a reduction of the catecholamine release thus improving cardiovascular and gastrointestinal manifestations and may prevent anatomical complications [52]. Although tumor progression is the most frequent cause of death from metastatic PCCs and PGGs, up to 30% of the deaths are due to hypertension and intestinal occlusion [51].

The diagnosis of pheochromocytoma is confirmed with high sensitivity (>90%) by elevated catecholamine metabolites (metanephrines) in plasma and, more commonly, by raised 24-h urinary excretion of fractionated metanephrines. However, plasma metanephrines have higher specificity compared with 24-h urine tests (ranging from 79% to 98% vs. 69% to 95%, respectively) [48, 49]. Many drugs can interfere with the testing of plasma/urine metanephrines leading to false-positive results and include acetaminophen, selective serotonin reuptake inhibitors, tricyclic antidepressants, monoamine oxidase inhibitors, and certain β-adrenergic and α-adrenergic blockers. These medications should be stopped for 10–14 days before testing if possible [48, 49]. If the medications cannot be stopped and the plasma/urine metanephrine levels are increased it is advised to perform imaging procedures [48].

Computed tomography or magnetic resonance imaging have a high sensitivity (90–95%) for detecting primary tumors and metastatic and extra-adrenal lesions larger than 1 cm. ^{18}F-fluorodeoxyglucose positron emission tomography (FDG-PET) is the most sensitive scintigraphic method for assessing metastatic PCCS and PGGs [51]. In addition, functional scintigraphy with ^{123}I-mIBG can be used to determine whether patients are candidates for targeted radiotherapy with ^{131}I-mIBG [48, 49, 51]. Given its high structural similarity with noradrenaline, mIBG is taken up by tumoral cells and causes radiation-induced cell death. ^{123}I-mIBG is superior to ^{131}I-mIBG for imaging in terms of physical properties, quality of images, and sensitivity (83–100%) and specificity (95–100%) [53]. Based on mIBG uptake on diagnostic imaging, around 50–60% patients with malignant PCCs and PGG are suitable for ^{131}I-mIBG therapy. The ideal candidates for mIBG therapy as a first-line therapy

are patients with significant tumor burden, slowly progressive disease, adequate mIBG uptake on diagnostic imaging, acceptable blood tests [49, 50]. Responses to therapy are generally better in patients with limited disease or soft-tissue metastases than in patients with bone metastases.

5.2.2 Indications

According to the EANM procedure guidelines [54], ^{131}I-mIBG therapy is indicated in all cases with inoperable PPCs and PPGs. Patients with metastatic disease, in course of progression and/or intractable pain, can be considered eligible for mIBG therapy [55–57]. Although nowadays, with the advent of peptide receptor radionuclide therapy (PRRNT), there might be some competition due to overlapping indications [58, 59], ^{131}I-mIBG therapy remains the most studied radionuclide therapy for these type of neuroendocrine tumors (Table 5.5).

^{131}I-mIBG therapy relies on the expression of norepinephrine transporters and vesicular monoamine transporters (VMAT) in tumors of neural crest origin [60–62]. Already after the initial imaging application in the 80s, it was clear that the majority of PPC/PPG concentrate ^{131}I-mIBG [63], which can be applied at higher doses for therapeutic purposes. However, not all forms of PPC/PPG concentrate mIBG. In case of malignant transformation or tumor dedifferentiation, in succinate dehydrogenase subunit B mutation (SDHB), von Hippel–Lindau syndrome, and in patients with dopamine-secreting forms, PPCs and PPGs can be mIBG-negative [64–66], hence the need for a baseline pre-radionuclide therapy assessment.

Therefore, the prerequisite for performing mIBG therapy is, in the first place, the documented mIBG-positivity of the lesions candidate to treatment as demonstrated on mIBG scan [54, 67]. The scintigraphy can be performed with either ^{123}I- or ^{131}I-mIBG, documenting an overall sensitivity and specificity of the modality in PPCs/PPGs between 83–100% and 95–100%, respectively [68, 69]. Tumors eligible for mIBG

Table 5.5 Summary of the studies investigating ^{131}I-mIBG therapy in pheochromocytoma (PCC) and paraganglioma (PPG)

Authors (year)	Patients (no.)	Tumor type	^{131}I-mIBG activity (mCi)	Cycles (no.)	Objective response	Biochemical response	Outcome
Shapiro et al. (1991)	28	PCC	97–301	1–6	7%	18%	Median PFS 18 months
Krempf et al. (1991)	15	PCC	78.4–250	1–11	33%	35%	Median TTP 36 months
Fischer et al. (1991)	14	PCC	64–210	1–6	14%	/	//
Lumborso et al. (1991)	11	PCC	100–200	1–6	15%	15%	Median OS 16 months
Schumberger et al. (1992)	20	PCC	100–200	1–6	15%	15%	Median OS 16 months
Bomanji et al. (1993)	5	2 PCC 2 PPG	83.7–300	1–7	60%	60%	Median OS >50 months
Loh et al. (1997)[a]	116	PCC	96–300	1-11	30%	45%	Relapse rate 45% in responder patients
Mukherjee et al. (2001)	15	8 PCC 7 PPG	100–300	1–7	40%	47%	5-year survival 85%
Rose et al. (2003)	12	6 PCC 6 PPG	386–866	1–3	33%	42%	Median response duration 34 months
Safford et al. (2003)	33	22 PCC 11 PPG	391+/−131	1–6	38%	60%	Median survival 4.7 years; 5-year survival 45%
Buskombe et al. (2005)	3	3 PCC 1 PPG	90–142	4–11	33%	/	Mean PFS 7.7 months
Sisson et al. (2006)	21	PCC	137–349	1–6	30%	/	5-year survival 70.5%
Fitzgerald et al. (2006)	30	11 PCC 19 PPG	557–1185	/	63%	/	Calculated 5-year survival 75%
Gedik et al. (2008)	19	12 PCC 7 PPG	100–700	1–10	47%	67%	Median PFS 24 months
Gonias et al. (2009)	50	15 PCC 34 PPG	492–1160	1–3	22%	66–74%	5-year survival 64%; 5-year EFS 47%
Shilkrut et al. (2010)	10	7 PCC 3 PPG	145.5	1–4	30%	50%	Median PFS 17.5 months
Navalkissor et al. (2010)	4	3 PCC 1 PPG	148.6–200	2–6	25%	/	Mean PFS 22 months
Castellani et al. (2010)	Group 1 (12/28)	4 PCC 8 PPG	124–149	7	33%	56%	Median response duration 1.9 years
	Group 2 (16/28)	11 PCC 5 PPG	200–350	2	31%	71.4%	Median response duration 3 years
Rachh et al. (2011)	12	8 PCC 4 PPG	/	1–5	8%	50%	Mean stability 29 months
Sze et al. (2013)	14	7 PCC 7 PPG	195	2	/	/	5-year survival 68%
Wakabayashi et al. (2013)	26	18 PCC 8 PPG	200	1–6	0%	35%	5-year survival 50%
Yoshinaga et al. (2014)	48	37 PCC 11 PPG	100–300	1–4	2%	0%	/
Rutherford et al. (2015)	22	10 PCC 12 PPG	135–305	1–5	19%	10%	Median survival after treatment start 11.1 years
Noto et al. (2018)	21	10 PCC 11 PPG	181–196	6	19%	80%	1-year survival 85.7% 2-year survival 61.9%

EFS event-free survival, *OS* overall survival, *PFS* progression-free survival, *TTP* time-to-progression
[a]This is a review article collecting data from 116 patients, 3 from the authors' own center and 113 reported in the literature from 1983 to 1996

therapy require a tumor uptake clearly above the background activity (visual) or with a lesion-to-background ratio >2 (*semiquantitative*) [55, 70]. Pretreatment scanning can be used in addition as an aid to calculate the dose and predict the level of uptake and retention of ^{131}I-mIBG during radionuclide therapy [56, 57, 71].

5.2.3 Patient Selection and Preparation

Once the inoperable/metastatic condition is determined and tumor lesions are documented to have an increased mIBG uptake, patients can be screened and prepared for radionuclide therapy. Patients eligible for mIBG therapy are preferably fit, with an acceptable performance status (Karnofsky >60; ECOG PS <2), a life expectancy superior to 3 months, adequate hematopoietic parameters, adequate renal function, and good liver function [54, 55, 70].

Before radionuclide therapy, all drugs interfering with intracellular mIBG uptake should be discontinued. Some of the most important competitors include tricyclic antidepressants, antiarrhythmics, α- and β-blockers, β-2 stimulants, some sympathomimetics, calcium channel blockers, antihistamines, opioid analgesics, reserpine, etc. The list of drugs comprises several classes of medication that are widely enumerated in the EANM guidelines [54].

For therapeutic purpose, mIBG is labelled with iodine-131, which can be found in the blood stream of the patient during treatment as free iodine. Free iodine can accumulate in the thyroid gland, resulting in direct damage to the organ with an increased risk of hypothyroidism. Therefore, it is mandatory to protect the gland by blocking iodine uptake before administering therapy with specific drugs, such as Lugol's solution, potassium iodine, or saturated solution of potassium iodide [72, 73]. Thyroid blockade should start 24–48 h before radionuclide therapy and be continued for 10–15 days after. Potassium perchlorate can also be used in combination with stable iodine to allow the wash out of the iodine-131 from the thyroid [74].

5.2.4 Radiopharmaceutical Preparation

For radionuclide therapy, mIBG is labelled with iodine-131. This isotope has a long half-life (8.02 days) and presents a high-to-medium energy beta emission (89.6% 0.606 MeV; 7.2% 0.333 MeV, 2% 0.247 MeV) [75], which allows for its therapeutic usage. The radionuclide is commercially supplied frozen in aqueous or glucose solutions, which has to be radiolabelled with iodine-131, up to a specific activity of 30–50 mCi/mg [70, 74]. This conventional method of preparation guarantees only one out of 2000 molecules of mIBG labelled with iodine-131. On counterpart, new ways for radiolabelling, also called no-carrier-added or carrier-free high-specific-activity preparations [76], have been implemented, allowing for a higher amount of iodinated mIBG molecules up to a specific activity of 2500 mCi/mg [77, 78].

Once prepared, ^{131}I-mIBG should be administered intravenously with a very slow infusion via a peripheral cannula or a central venous line. After the infusion, the line should be flushed very slowly too to avoid hypertensive crises. Blood pressure and other vital signs should be monitored during the infusion and the recovery following the administration [54].

5.2.5 Treatment Schedules

The therapeutic regimens with ^{131}I-mIBG, comprising number of doses and administered activities, can be quite variegate. While the EANM guideline reports single doses ranging from 100 mCi to 300 mCi [54], in literature the administered activities range from 64 mCi to 1165 mCi (Table 5.5). The computation of these activities can be performed either empirically, by using fixed doses or fixed activities per body weight, or following dosimetric estimation [74, 79]. The later one is to be preferred, since it is more reproducible and can maintain the amount of activity within the dose constrain levels. Along with dose levels, also the number of doses/cycles of radionuclide therapy is variable. Most treatment schedules consider multiple doses of ^{131}I-mIBG (range 1–11), administered every 3–6 months [79]. The regimen chosen for the treatment should have in all cases the intent to give a sufficient amount of dose to the tumor lesions to obtain a biochemical or objective response. According to the reported data, an estimated dose of 150 Gy can be considered as advisable for this purpose [79].

5.2.6 Results

Based on the indications, the majority of patients with PPC/PPG candidate to radionuclide therapy are metastatic, with either progressive or symptomatic disease. Hence, one of the most desirable effects required from MIBG therapy is tumor reduction, with biochemical response and clinical release of the symptoms. A complete response to therapy, however, is less frequent than imagined since published data report quite low rates, ranging from 0% to 18% [74, 79]. Hence, objective and biochemical responses are more commonly considered when assessing the efficacy of mIBG therapy. Depending on the administered activity and the number of doses, objective response varies from 0% to 63% [80, 81] (Fig. 5.5) with the majority of the studies reporting responses below 50% [79] (Table 5.5). mIBG therapy has instead a more robust impact on symptom relief and palliation related to catecholamine excretion. In this context, particularly in multiple-dose schedules, the benefit from ^{131}I-mIBG is around 50% to 85% [82, 83].

The introduction of high-dose regimens and with the advent of high-specific-activity ^{131}I-mIBG, the objective and biochemical response rates are expected to increase. In case of high-dose therapy, objective response rates are reported in up to 30% of the patients, symptomatic responses can reach

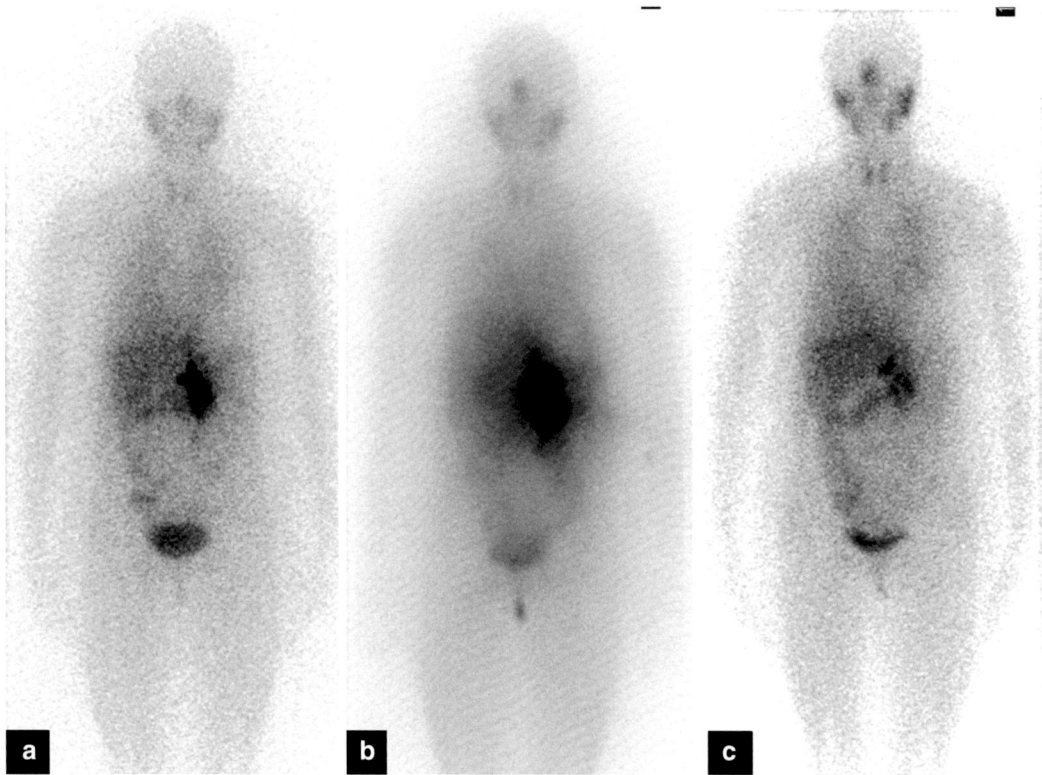

Fig. 5.5 Sixty-four years female affected by unresectable abdominal metastases by PCC able to concentrate mIBG (**a**) Patients underwent ^{131}I-mIBG therapy (300 mCi) and post-therapeutic whole body scintigraphy (**b**) confirmed the abdominal sites of disease. Seven months later, a diagnostic ^{123}I-mIBG whole body scintigraphy (**c**) demonstrated partial metabolic response to treatment. *NB* neuroblastoma, *PCC* pheochromocytoma

92%, while biochemical responses can be seen in up to 74% of the patients [84, 85]. Recently, the results of a Phase I clinical trial on high-specific-activity mIBG therapy, have been reported by Noto et al. [86]. In this study, when applying a maximal tolerable activity of 296 MBq/Kg, the best biochemical responses were observed in 80% and 64% of patients for chromogranin A and metanephrines, respectively. Whereas objective response was documented on RECIST (Response Evaluation Criteria in Solid Tumors) criteria as partial tumor regression in 19 patients (21% of the cases).

The responses obtained with the different regimens mentioned above can have quite variable duration. Median duration of response is reported between 1.9 and 3 years [87], with a median progression-free survival reported between 17.5 and 24 months [83, 88]. The survival benefit is more difficult to determine, although there are data suggesting a longer OS for patients treated with higher single doses (400 mCi) and in patients showing a symptomatic response and biochemical improvement after therapy [79]. Reported overall survival ranges from 16 months to more than 50 months [89–91], with a 5-year survival rate ranging from 45% to 85% [82, 85].

5.2.7 Side Effects and Complications

[131]I-mIBG therapy can be associated with early and delayed side effects and toxicities. Some of them can be temporary and of limited clinical relevance, such as asthenia, nausea and vomiting, transitory myelosuppression or hematologic toxicities, salivary gland tenderness and short-term salivary dysfunction, pulmonary adverse effects, hypertensive crises, etc. Others can be more dramatic or leave long-term consequences, comprising bone marrow depression, deterioration of renal function, ARDS (acute respiratory distress syndrome) and bronchiolitis obliterans, myelodysplasia, up to sparse secondary tumors or leukemia. Within the delayed toxicities, we can find also hypothyroidism and hypogonadism, the former depending principally on the quality

of thyroid blockade [54, 74]. With the introduction of high-specific-activity mIBG, allowing for a better targeting of the tumor lesions, it might be possible to reduce the amount of side effects and toxicities. Although we need more data, we have already evidence of lower incidence for some side effects, such as nausea, vomiting, and hypertension [79].

5.3 Dosimetric Approach to Neuroblastoma and Pheocromocytoma to Improve Safety and Effectiveness

In the ^{131}I-mIBG treatments of NB and PCCs, bone marrow toxicity limits the amount of administered activity and the therapeutic tumor dose. Since the dose to the bone marrow is a measure of hematologic toxicity, ideally bone marrow dosimetry for a specific patient should be performed prior to therapy, so that the total administered activity can be prescribed accordingly. To calculate the bone marrow absorbed dose it is necessary to carry out a series of blood samples and of whole body counts. Therefore, calculating the bone marrow absorbed dose can be difficult, especially in pediatric patients. In practice, the whole body is introduced as a surrogate for bone marrow, and then, the whole body dosimetry, more easily feasible, is used instead of bone marrow dosimetry. Indeed, Matthay et al. [92] demonstrated in 42 patients with neuroblastoma that the absorbed bone marrow correlates with the whole body absorbed dose. Furthermore, Buckley et al. [93] showed that whole body absorbed dose is a most accurate predictor of hematological toxicity in NB patients treated with ^{131}I-mIBG therapy. Then the prescription of administered activity based on whole-body absorbed dose allows personalized treatment according to an individual's hematologic toxicity.

George et al. [94] calculated in 25 children affected by NB a mean whole body absorbed dose per unit activity equal to 0.22 Gy/GBq. Therefore, for an administered activity of 11.1 GBq (300 mCi) the whole body dose is

2.4 Gy. This value is in good agreement with other studies on this issue. Matthay et al. [95] in 15 patients, Gaze et al. [96] in 8 patients, and Bolster et al. [97] in 7 patients calculated mean values of 0.23, 0.26, and 0.25 Gy/GBq, respectively. By contrast, higher values have been evaluated in children affected by NB by other authors: Fielding et al. [98] in 25 patients calculated a mean whole body absorbed of 0.33 Gy/GBq, while Sudbrock et al. [99] in 14 patients and Monsieurs et al. [100] in 6 patients values equal to 0.31 and 0.37 Gy/GBq, respectively. The differences between the whole body absorbed dose values in NB patients reported in these studies could be related to the different residual tumor burden. Indeed, the whole body kinetics is heavily influenced by that of the tumor.

Different studies conducted in adults affected by PPC showed comparable body-absorbed dose values. Tristam et al. [101] in 12 patients calculated a mean value of 0.12 Gy/GBq, similarly Sudbrock et al. [99] and Ertl et al. [102] in 4 and 3 patients, calculated a mean value equal to 0.14 and 0.11 Gy/GBq, respectively. The significant difference between the whole body absorbed dose values in NB and in PPC is related to the different mass of the patients studied. In NB studies, all patients were children, while in those with PPCs all patients included were adults.

Buckley et al. [103] demonstrated in NB patients that there is no correlation between the absorbed dose by the whole body and that by the tumor. Indeed, tumor burden varies significantly and whole body absorbed dose is largely determined by kidney function. Moreover, Matthay et al. [92] in a large number of patients affected by NB demonstrated the existence of a correlation between the tumor absorbed dose for values >10 Gy and the tumor volume decrease. In this context, tumor dosimetry appears to be the most important index able to predict the outcome after ^{131}I-mIBG therapy. Furthermore the knowledge of the absorbed dose by the tumor as well as by organs would also allow to combine ^{131}I-mIBG therapy with external beam radiotherapy [104] in order to obtain higher value of tumor absorbed dose not achievable with ^{131}I-mIBG alone. Thus, an ideal scenario for a pretreatment investiga-

tion would include both whole body and tumor dosimetry. To calculate the whole body absorbed dose before therapy it is necessary to evaluate the clearance of ^{131}I-mIBG tracer making measurements over time using a whole body counter. Instead, for tumor dosimetry the ^{123}I-mIBG is most suitable, since it allows to obtain better scintigraphic images compared to ^{131}I-mIBG, that is because the energy of the γ-ray emission of [123]I (159 keV) is close to the ideal for imaging using gamma cameras.

The few studies that calculated the tumor absorbed dose in NB and PCC showed that it varies widely. This is due to the large variability between tumors, also within the same typology of disease, regarding uptake and effective half-life. Sudbrock et al. [99] calculated in 24 tumors (16 neuroblastoma and 8 pheochromocytoma) a mean tumor absorbed dose of 3.0 Gy/GBq (range 1.1–5.8 Gy/GBq), while Tristam et al. [101] in 20 tumors (4 NB and 16 PCC) calculated a mean tumor absorbed dose of 2.2 Gy/GBq (range 0.04–20.0 Gy/GBq). Fielding et al. [98] in 7 NB tumors in children evaluated an absorbed dose value of 5.4 Gy/GBq (range 0.2–16.6 Gy/GBq), whereas Koral et al. [105] in 7 pheochromocytoma tumors in adults a value of 9.2 Gy/GBq (range 2.2–21.6 Gy/GBq).

Therefore, for an administered activity equal to 11.1 GBq the tumor absorbed dose can range widely from few to hundreds of Grays.

Since ^{131}I-mIBG is cleared through the urine, the bladder could receive during treatment a high radiation exposure such as to limit the administered activity. Fielding et al. [98] in 5 children affected by NB without bladder catheters calculated a mean bladder wall absorbed dose equal to 3.1 Gy/GBq, and in 23 children a mean bone marrow absorbed dose of 0.34 Gy/GBq. Bolster et al. [97] in 7 children affected by NB without bladder catheters calculated a much lower mean bladder wall absorbed dose compared to Fielding et al. [98] equal to 0.76 Gy/GBq. This huge difference is due to the fact that the wall bladder absorbed dose during treatment with ^{131}I-mIBG is strongly dependent on hydration and renal function of the patient. Koral et al. [106] and Matthay et al. [95] in 7 and 15 children with NB evaluated a mean liver absorbed dose of 0.79 and 0.92 Gy/GBq, respectively.

In conclusion, a personalized dosimetry, scheduled before ^{131}I-mIBG, able to predict the dose to the bone marrow and to the tumor, seems to be an important starting point to both select the correct activity and limit toxicities.

References

1. Monclair T, Brodeur GM, Ambros PF, Brisse HJ, Cecchetto G, Holmes K, et al. The International Neuroblastoma Risk Group (INRG) staging system: an INRG task force report. J Clin Oncol. 2009;27:298–303.
2. Park JR, Eggert A, Caron H. Neuroblastoma: biology, prognosis, and treatment. Hematol Oncol Clin North Am. 2010;24:65–86.
3. Brodeur GM. Neuroblastoma: biological insights into a clinical enigma. Nat Rev Cancer. 2003;3:203–16.
4. Rohrer T, Trachsel D, Engelcke G, Hammer J. Congenital central hypoventilation syndrome associated with Hirschsprung's disease and neuroblastoma: case of multiple neurocristopathies. Pediatr Pulmonol. 2002;33:71–6.
5. Trigg RM, Turner SD. ALK in neuroblastoma: biological and therapeutic implications. Cancers. 2018;10:10.
6. Cohn SL, Pearson AD, London WB, Monclair T, Ambros PF, Brodeur GM, et al. The International Neuroblastoma Risk Group (INRG) classification system: an INRG task force report. J Clin Oncol. 2009;27:289–97.
7. Beiske K, Burchill SA, Cheung IY, Hiyama E, Seeger RC, Cohn SL, et al. Consensus criteria for sensitive detection of minimal neuroblastoma cells in bone marrow, blood and stem cell preparations by immunocytology and QRT-PCR: recommendations by the International Neuroblastoma Risk Group Task Force. Br J Cancer. 2009;100:1627–37.
8. Ambros PF, Ambros IM, Brodeur GM, Haber M, Khan J, Nakagawara A, et al. International consensus for neuroblastoma molecular diagnostics: report from the International Neuroblastoma Risk Group (INRG) Biology Committee. Br J Cancer. 2009;100:1471–82.
9. Matthay KK, Shulkin B, Ladenstein R, Michon J, Giammarile F, Lewington V, et al. Criteria for evaluation of disease extent by (123) I-metaiodobenzylguanidine scans in neuroblastoma: a report for the International Neuroblastoma Risk Group (INRG) task force. Br J Cancer. 2010;102:1319–26.
10. Brisse HJ, McCarville MB, Granata C, Krug KB, Wootton-Gorges SL, Kanegawa K, et al. Guidelines for imaging and staging of neuroblastic tumors: consensus report from the International Neuroblastoma Risk Group project. Radiology. 2011;261:243–57.
11. Maris JM. Recent advances in neuroblastoma. N Engl J Med. 2010;362:2202–11.
12. Pinto NR, Applebaum MA, Volchenboum SL, Matthay KK, London WB, Ambros PF, et al. Advances in risk classification and treatment-strategies for neuroblastoma. J Clin Oncol. 2015;33:3008–17.
13. Canete A, Gerrard M, Rubie H, Castel V, Di Cataldo A, Munzer C, et al. Poor survival for infants with MYCN-amplified metastatic neuroblastoma despite intensified treatment: the International Society of Paediatric Oncology European Neuroblastoma Experience. J Clin Oncol. 2009;27:1014–9.
14. Garaventa A, Boni L, Lo Piccolo MS, Tonini GP, Gambini C, Mancini A, et al. Localized unresectable neuroblastoma: results of treatment based on clinical prognostic factors. Ann Oncol. 2002;13:956–64.
15. Tanabe M, Takahashi H, Ohnuma N, Iwai J, Yoshida H. Evaluation of bone marrow metastasis of neuroblastoma and changes after chemotherapy by MRI. Med Pediatr Oncol. 1993;21:54–9.
16. Wilson JS, Gains JE, Moroz V, Wheatley K, Gaze MN. A systematic review of 131I-meta iodobenzylguanidine molecular radiotherapy for neuroblastoma. Eur J Cancer. 2014;50:801–15.
17. Castellani MR, Scarale A, Lorenzoni A, Maccauro M, Balaguer Guill J, Luksch R. Treatment with 131I-MIBG (indications, procedures and results) Chapter 19. In: Bombardieri E, editor. Clinical applications of nuclear medicine targeted therapy. Basingstoke: Springer Nature; 2018.
18. Shulkin BL, Shapiro B, Francis IR, et al. Primary extra-adrenal pheochromocytoma: positive I-123 MIBG imaging with negative I-131 MIBG imaging. Clin Nucl Med. 1986;11:851–4.
19. Brodeur GM, Pritchard J, Berthold F, Carlsen NL, Castel V, Castelberry RP, et al. Revisions of the international criteria for neuroblastoma diagnosis, staging, and response to treatment. J Clin Oncol. 1993;11:1466–77.
20. Schmidt M, Simon T, Hero B, et al. The prognostic impact of functional imaging with (123)ImIBGin patients with stage 4 neuroblastoma. 1 year of age on a high-risk treatment protocol: results of the German neuroblastoma trial NB97. Eur J Cancer. 2008;44:1552–8.
21. Boubaker A, Bischof Delaloye A. MIBG scintigraphy for the diagnosis and follow-up of children with neuroblastoma. Q J Nucl Med Mol Imaging. 2008;52:388–402.
22. Kushner BH, Yeh SD, Kramer K, et al. Impact of metaiodobenzylguanidine scintigraphy on assessing response of high-risk neuroblastoma to doseintensive induction chemotherapy. J Clin Oncol. 2003;21:1082–6.
23. Matthay KK, Edeline V, Lumbroso J, et al. Correlation of early metastatic response by 123I-metaiodobenzylguanidine scintigraphy with

overall response and event-free survival in stage IV neuroblastoma. J Clin Oncol. 2003;21:2486–91.

24. Matthay KK, Maris JM, Schleiermacher G, Nakagawara A, Mackall CL, Diller L, Weiss WA. Neuroblastoma. Nat Rev Dis Primers. 2016; 2:16078.

25. de Kraker J, Hoefnagel KA, Verschuur AC, van Eck B, van Santen HM, Caron HN, et al. Iodine-131-metaiodobenzylguanidine as initial induction therapy in stage 4 neuroblastoma patients over 1 year of age. Eur J Cancer. 2008;44:551–6.

26. Mastrangelo S, Rufini V, Ruggiero A, Di Giannatale A, Riccard R. Treatment of advanced neuroblastoma in children over 1 year of age: the critical role of 131I-metaiodobenzylguanidine combined with chemotherapy in a rapid induction regimen. Pediatr Blood Cancer. 2011;56:1032–40.

27. Klingebiel T, Bader P, Bares R, Beck J, Hero B, Jurgens H, et al. Treatment of neuroblastoma stage 4 with 131I-meta-iodo-benzylguanidine, high-dose chemotherapy and immunotherapy. A pilot study. Eur J Cancer. 1998;34(9):1398–402.

28. Giammarile F, Chiti A, Lassmann M, Brans B, Flux G, EANM. EANM procedure guidelines for 131I-meta-iodobenzylguanidine (131I-mIBG) therapy. Eur J Nucl Med Mol Imaging. 2008;35:1039–47.

29. Wilson JS, Gains JE, Moroz V, Wheatley K, Gaze MN. A systematic review of 131I-meta iodobenzylguanidine molecular radiotherapy for neuroblastoma. Eur J Cancer. 2014;50:801–15.

30. DuBois SG, Messina J, Maris JM, Huberty J, Glidden DV, Veatch J, et al. Hematologic toxicity of high-dose iodine-131-metaiodobenzylguanidine therapy for advanced neuroblastoma. J Clin Oncol. 2004;22:2452–60.

31. Hutchinson RJ, Sisson JC, Shapiro B, Miser JS, Normole D, Shulkin BL, et al. 131-I-metaiodobenzylguanidine treatment in patients with refractory advanced neuroblastoma. Am J Clin Oncol. 1992;15:226–32.

32. Matthay KK, Yanik G, Messina J, Quach A, Huberty J, Cheng SC, et al. Phase II study on the effect of disease sites, age, and prior therapy on response to iodine-131-metaiodobenzylguanidine therapy in refractory neuroblastoma. J Clin Oncol. 2007;25:1054–60.

33. Klingebiel T, Feine U, Treuner J, Reuland P, Handgretinger R, Niethammer D, et al. Treatment of neuroblastoma with [131I]metaiodobenzylguanidine: long-term results in 25 patients. J Nucl Biol Med. 1991;35:216–9.

34. Matthay KK, Quach A, Huberty J, Franc BL, Hawkins RA, Jackson H, et al. Iodine-131-metaiodobenzylguanidine double infusion with autologous stem-cell rescue for neuroblastoma: a new approaches to neuroblastoma therapy phase I study. J Clin Oncol. 2009;27:1020–5.

35. Johnson K, McGlynn B, Saggio J, Baniewicz D, Zhuang H, Maris JM, et al. Safety and efficacy of tandem 131I-metaiodobenzylguanidine infusions in relapsed/refractory neuroblastoma. Pediatr Blood Cancer. 2011;57:1124–9.

36. Matthay KK, Tan JC, Villablanca JG, Yanik GA, Veatch J, Franc B, et al. Phase I dose escalation of iodine-131-metaiodobenzylguanidine with myeloablative chemotherapy and autologous stem-cell transplantation in refractory neuroblastoma: a new approaches to Neuroblastoma Therapy Consortium Study. J Clin Oncol. 2006;24:500–6.

37. Miano M, Garaventa A, Pizzitola MR, Piccolo MS, Dallorso S, Villavecchia GP, et al. Megatherapy combining 131I metaiodobenzylguanidine and high-dose chemotherapy with haematopoietic progenitor cell rescue for neuroblastoma. Bone Marrow Transplant. 2001;27:571–4.

38. Schmidt M, Simon T, Hero B, Eschner W, Dietlein M, Sudbrock F, et al. Is there a benefit of 131I-MIBG therapy in the treatment of children with stage 4 neuroblastoma? A retrospective evaluation of The German Neuroblastoma Trial NB97 and implications for The German Neuroblastoma Trial NB2004. Nucl Med. 2006;45:145–51.

39. Ehninger G, Klingebiel T, Kumbier I, Schuler U, Feine U, Treuner J, Waller HD. Stability and pharmacokinetics of m-[131I]iodobenzylguanidine in patients. Cancer Res. 1987;47:6147–9.

40. Parisi MT, Eslamy H, Park JR, Shulkin BL, Yanik GA. 131I-metaiodobenzylguanidine theranostics in neuroblastoma:historical perspectives; practical applications. Semin Nucl Med. 2016;46:184–202.

41. Matthay KK, DeSantes K, Hasegawa B, et al. Phase I dose escalation of I-131-metaiodobenzylguanidine with autologous bone marrow support in refractory neuroblastoma. J Clin Oncol. 1998;16:229–36.

42. Matthay KK, DeSantes K, Hasegawa B, Huberty J, Hattner RS, Ablin A, et al. Phase I dose escalation of 131I-metaiodobenzylguanidine with autologous bone marrow support in refractory neuroblastoma. J Clin Oncol. 1998;16:229–36.

43. Bleeker G, Schoot RA, Caron HN, de Kraker J, Hoefnagel CA, van Eck BL, Tytgat GA. Toxicity of upfront 131I-metaiodobenzylguanidine (131I-MIBG) therapy in newly diagnosed neuroblastoma patients: a retrospective analysis. Eur J Nucl Med Mol Imaging. 2013;40(11):1711–7.

44. Van Santen HM, de Kraker J, van Eck BLF, de Vijlder JJM, Vulsma T. Improved radiation protection of the thyroid gland with thyroxine, methimazole, and potassiumiodide during diagnostic and therapeutic use of radiolabeled metaiodobenzylguanidine in children with neuroblastoma. Cancer. 2003;98:389–96.

45. Clement SC, van Rijn RR, van Eck-Smit BL, van Trotsenburg AS, Caron HN, Tytgat GA, van Santen HM. Long-term efficacy of current thyroid prophylaxis and future perspectives on thyroid protection during 131I-metaiodobenzylguanidine treatment in children with neuroblastoma. Eur J Nucl Med Mol Imaging. 2015;42:706–15.

46. Kayano D, Kinuya S. Iodine-131 metaiodo-benzylguanidine therapy for neuroblastoma: reports so far and future perspective. ScientificWorldJournal. 2015;2015:189135. https://doi.org/10.1155/2015/189135.

47. Garaventa A, Gambini C, Villavecchia G, et al. Secondmalignancies in children with neuroblastoma after combined treatment with 131I-metaiodobenzylguanidine. Cancer. 2003; 97(5):1332–8.

48. Fishbein L. Pheochromocytoma and paraganglioma: genetics, diagnosis, and treatment. Hematol Oncol Clin North Am. 2016;30:135–50. https://doi.org/10.1016/j.hoc.2015.09.006.

49. Gunawardane KPT, Grossman A. Pheochromocytoma and paraganglioma. Adv Exp Med Biol. 2017;956:239–59. https://doi.org/10.1007/5584, Springer International Publishing Switzerland.

50. Adjallé R, Plouin PF, Pacak K, Lehnert H. Treatment of malignant pheochromocytoma. Horm Metab Res. 2009;4:687–96. https://doi.org/10.1055/s-0029-1231025.

51. Baudin E, Habra MA, Deschamps F, Cote G, Dumont F, Cabanillas M, Arfi-Roufe J, Berdelou A, Moon B, Al Ghuzlan A, Patel S, Leboulleux S, Jimenez C. Therapy of endocrine disease: treatment of malignant pheochromocytoma and paraganglioma. Eur J Endocrinol. 2014;171:R111–22. https://doi.org/10.1530/EJE-14-0113.

52. Jimenez P, Tatsui C, Jessop A, Thosani S, Jimenez C. Treatment for malignant pheochromocytomas and paragangliomas: 5 years of progress. Curr Oncol Rep. 2017;19:83. https://doi.org/10.1007/s11912-017-0643-0.

53. Parenti G, Zampetti B, Rapizzi E, Ercolino T, Giachè V, Mannelli M. Updated and new perspectives on diagnosis, prognosis, and therapy of malignant pheochromocytoma/paraganglioma. J Oncol. 2012;2012:872713. https://doi.org/10.1155/2012/872713.

54. Giammarile F, Chiti A, Lassmann M, et al. EANM procedure guidelins for 131I-metiodobenzylguanidine (131I-mIBG) therapy. Eur J Nucl Med Mol Imaging. 2008;35:1039–47.

55. Carrasquillo JA, Pandit-Taskar N, Chen CC. Radionuclide therapy of adrenal tumors. J Surg Oncol. 2012;106:632–42.

56. Pasieka JL, McEwan AJB, Rorstad O. The palliative role ofI-131-MIBG and In-111-octreotide therapy in patients withmetastatic progressive neuroendocrine neoplasms. Surgery. 2004;136:1218–26.

57. Nguyen C, Faraggi M, Giraudet AL, et al. Long-term efficacyof radionuclide therapy in patients with disseminated neuroendocrinetumors uncontrolled by conventional therapy. J Nucl Med. 2004;45:1660–8.

58. Zaknun JJ, Bodei L, Mueller-Brand J, et al. The joint IAEA, EANM, and SNMMI practical guidance on peptide receptor radionuclide therapy (PRRNT)

in neuroendocrine tumours. Eur J Nucl Med Mol Imaging. 2013;40:800–16.

59. Saveanu A, Muresan M, De Micco C, et al. Expression of somatostatin receptors, dopamine D-2 receptors, noradrenaline transporters, and vesicular monoamine transporters in 52 pheochromocytomas and paragangliomas. Endocr Relat Cancer. 2011;18:287–300.

60. Sisson JC, Shapiro B, Beierwaltes WH, et al. Radio pharmaceutical treatment of malignant pheochromocytoma. J Nucl Med. 1984;25:197–206.

61. Huynh TT, Pacak K, Brouwers FM, et al. Different expression of catecholamine transporters in phaeochromocytomas from patients with Von Hippel-Lindau syndrome and multiple endocrine neoplasia type 2. Eur J Endocrinol. 2005;153:551–63.

62. Fottner C, Helisch A, Anlauf M, et al. 6-18F-fluoro-idihydroxyphenylalanine positron emission tomography is superior to 123I-metaiodobenzyl-guanidine scintigraphy in the detection of extra-adrenal and hereditary pheochromocytomas and paragangliomas: with vesicular monoamine transporter expression. J Clin Endocrinol Metab. 2010;95:2800–10.

63. Dahia PL. Pheochromocytoma and paraganglioma pathogenesis: learning fromgenetic heterogeneity. Nat Rev Cancer. 2014;14:108–19.

64. Dubois LA, Gray DK. Dopamine-secreting pheochromocytomas: in search of a syndrome. World J Surg. 2005;29:909–13.

65. Kaji P, Carrasquillo JA, Linehan WM, et al. The role of 6-[18F]fluorodopaminepositron emission tomography in the localization of adrenal pheochromocytomaassociated with von Hippel-Lindau syndrome. Eur J Endocrinol. 2007;156:483–7.

66. Parenti G, Zampetti B, Rapizzi E, et al. Updated and new perspectices on diagnosis, prognosis, and therapy of malignant pheochromocytoma/paraganglioma. J Oncol. 2012;2012:872713.

67. van Berkel A, Rao JU, Lenders JWM, et al. Semiquantitative I-123- metaiodobenzylguanidine scintigraphy to distinguish pheochromocy- toma and paraganglioma from physiologic adrenal uptake and its correlation with genotype-dependent expression of catecholamine trans- porters. J Nucl Med. 2015;56:839–46.

68. Ilias I, Pacak K. Current approaches and recommended algorithm for the diagnostic localization of pheochromocytoma. J Clin Endocrinol Metab. 2004;89:479–91.

69. Shulkin BL, Ilias I, Sisson JC, Pacak K. Current trends in functional imaging of pheochromocytomas and paragangliomas. Ann N Y Acad Sci. 2006;1073:374–82.

70. Gonias S, Goldsby R, Matthay KK, et al. Phase II study of high-dose I-131 metaiodobenzylguanidine therapy for patients with metastatic pheochromocytoma and paraganglioma. J Clin Oncol. 2009;27:4162–8.

71. Shapiro B, Sisson JC, Lloyd R, et al. Malignant pheochromocytoma: clinical, biochemical and

scintigraphic characterization. Clin Endocrinol. 1984;20:189–203.

72. Sternthal E, Lipworth L, Stanley B, et al. Suppression of thyroid radioiodine uptake by various doses of stable iodide. N Engl J Med. 1980;303:1083–1088 55.

73. Zanzonico PB, Becker DV. Effects of time of administration and dietary iodine levels on potassium iodide (KI) blockade of thyroid irradiation by I-131 from radioactive fallout. Health Phys. 2000;78:660–667 56.

74. Carrasquillo JA, Pandiut-Taskar N, Chen CC. I-131 metaiodobenzylguanidine therapy of pheochromocytoma and paraganglioma. Semin Nucl Med. 2016;46:203–14.

75. Lopci E, Chiti A, Castellani MR, et al. Matched pairs dosimetry: 124I/131I metaiodobenzylguanidine and 124I/131/ and 86Y/90/Y antibodies. Eur J Nucl Med Mol Imaging. 2011;38(Suppl 1):S28–40.

76. Coleman RE, Stubbs JB, Barrett JA, et al. Radiation dosimetry, pharmacokinetics, and safety of ultra-trace (TM) iobenguane I-131 in patients with malignant pheochromocytoma/paraganglioma or metastatic carcinoid. Cancer Biother Radiopharm. 2009;24:469–75.

77. Mairs RJ, Gaze MN, Watson DG, et al. Carrier-freeI-131 metaiodobenzylguanidine—comparison of production from meta-diazobenzylguanidine and from meta-trimethylsilylbenzylguanidine. Nucl Med Commun. 1994;15:268–74.

78. Vaidyanathan G, Affleck DJ, Zalutsky MR. No-carrier-added synthesis of a 4-methyl-substituted meta-iodobenzylguanidine analogue. Appl Radiat Isot. 2005;62:435–440 40.

79. Pandit-Taskar N, Modak S. Norepinephrine transporter as a target for imagingand therapy. J Nucl Med. 2017;58(Suppl 2):39S–53S.

80. Wakabayashi H, Taki J, Inaki A, et al. Prognostic values of initial responses to low-dose I-131-MIBG therapy in patients with malignant pheochromocytoma and paraganglioma. Ann Nucl Med. 2013;27:839–46.

81. Fitzgerald PA, Goldsby RE, Huberty JP, et al. Malignant pheochromocytomas and paragangliomas. A phse II study of therapy with high-dose 131-metaiodobenzylguanidine (131I-MIBG). Ann N Y Acad Sci. 2006;1073:465–90.

82. Safford SD, Coleman E, Gockerman JP, et al. Iodine-131 metaiodoben- zylguanidine is an effective treatment formalignant pheochromocytoma and paraganglioma. Surgery. 2003;134:956–62.

83. Shilkrut M, Bar-Deroma R, Bar-Sela G, et al. Low-dose iodine-131 metaiodobenzylguanidine therapy for patients with malignant pheochromocytoma and paraganglioma single center experience. Am J Clin Oncol. 2010;33:79–82.

84. Pathirana AA, Vinjamuri S, Byrne C, Ghaneh P, Vora J, Poston GJ. I-131-MIBG radionuclide therapy is safe and cost-effective in the control of symptoms of the carcinoid syndrome. Eur J Surg Oncol. 2001;27:404–8.

85. Mukherjee JJ, Kaltsas GA, Islam N, et al. Treatment of metastatic carcinoid tumours, phaeochromocytoma, paraganglioma andmedullary carcinoma of the thyroid with I-131-meta-iodobenzylguanidine (I-131- MIBG). Clin Endocrinol. 2001;55:47–60.

86. Noto RB, Pryma DA, Jensen J, et al. Phase 1 study of high-specific-activity I-131 MIBG for metastatic and/or recurrent pheochromocytoma or paraganglioma. J Clin Endocrinol Metab. 2018 Jan 1;103:213–20.

87. Castellani MR, Seghezzi S, Chiesa C, et al. I-131-MIBG treatment of pheochromocytoma: low versus intermediate activity regimens of therapy. Q J Nucl Med Mol Imaging. 2010;54:100–13.

88. Gedik GK, Hoefnagel CA, Bais E, et al. 131I-MIBG therapyinmetastatic phaeochromocytoma and paraganglioma. Eur J Nucl Med Mol Imaging. 2008;35:725–33.

89. Lumbroso J, Schlumberger M, Tenenbaum F, et al. 131I Metaiodobenzylguanidine therapy in 20 patients with malignant pheochromocytoma. J Nucl Biol Med. 1991;35:288–91.

90. Schlumberger M, Gicquel C, Lumbroso J, et al. Malignant pheochromocytoma—clinical, biological, histologic and therapeutic data in a series of 20 patients with distant metastases. J Endocrinol Invest. 1992;15:631–42.

91. Bomanji J, Britton KE, Ur E, et al. Treatment of malignant pheochro- mocytoma, paraganglioma and carcinoid-tumors with I-131 metaiodo- benzylguanidine. Nucl Med Commun. 1993;14:856–61.

92. Matthay KK, Panina C, Huberty J, Price D, Glidden DV, Tang HR, Hawkins RA, Veatch J, Hasegawa B. Correlation of tumor and whole-body dosimetry with tumor response and toxicity in refractory neuroblastoma treated with (131)I-MIBG. J Nucl Med. 2001;42:1713–21.

93. Buckley SE, Chittenden SJ, Saran FH, Meller ST, Flux GD. Whole-body dosimetry for individualized treatment planning of 131I-MIBG radionuclide therapy for neuroblastoma. J Nucl Med. 2009;50:1518–24.

94. George SL, Falzone N, Chittenden S, Kirk SJ, Lancaster D, Vaidya SJ, Mandeville H, Saran F, Pearson AD, Du Y, Meller ST, Denis-Bacelar AM, Flux GD. Individualized 131I-mIBG therapy in the management of refractory and relapsed neuroblastoma. Nucl Med Commun. 2016;37:466–72.

95. Matthay KK, Weiss B, Villablanca JG, Maris JM, Yanik GA, Dubois SG, Stubbs J, Groshen S, Tsao-Wei D, Hawkins R, Jackson H, Goodarzian F, Daldrup-Link H, Panigrahy A, Towbin A, Shimada H, Barrett J, Lafrance N, Babich J. Dose escalation study of no-carrier-added 131I-metaiodobenzylguanidine for relapsed or refractory neuroblastoma: new approaches to neuroblastoma therapy consortium trial. J Nucl Med. 2012;53:1155–63.

96. Gaze MN, Chang YC, Flux GD, Mairs RJ, Saran FH, Meller ST. Feasibility of dosimetry-based high-dose 131I-meta-iodobenzylguanidine with topotecan as a radiosensitizer in children with metastatic

neuroblastoma. Cancer Biother Radiopharm. 2005;20:195–9.

97. Bolster A, Hilditch T, Wheldon T, Gaze M, Barrett A. Dosimetric considerations in 131I-MIBG therapy for neuroblastoma in children. Br J Radiol. 1995;68:481–90.

98. Fielding SL, Flower MA, Ackery D, Kemshead JT, Lashford LS, Lewis I. Dosimetry of iodine 131 metaiodobenzylguanidine for treatment of resistant neuroblastoma: results of a UK study. Eur J Nucl Med. 1991;18:308–16.

99. Sudbrock F, Schmidt M, Simon T, Eschner W, Berthold F, Schicha H. Dosimetry for 131I-MIBG therapies in metastatic neuroblastoma, phaeochromocytoma and paraganglioma. Eur J Nucl Med Mol Imaging. 2010;37:1279–90.

100. Monsieurs M, Brans B, Bacher K, Dierckx R, Thierens H. Patient dosimetry for 131I-MIBG therapy for neuroendocrine tumours based on 123I-MIBG scans. Eur J Nucl Med Mol Imaging. 2002;29:1581–7.

101. Tristam M, Alaamer A, Fleming J, Lewington V, Zivanovic M. Iodine-131-metaiodobenzylguanidine dosimetry in cancer therapy. J Nucl Med. 1996; 37:1058–63.

102. Ertl S, Deckart H, Blottner A, Tautz M. Radiopharmacokinetics and radiation absorbed dose calculations from 131I-meta-iodobenzylguanidine (131I-MIBG). Nucl Med Commun. 1987;8:643–53.

103. Buckley SE, Saran FH, Gaze MN, Chittenden S, Partridge M, Lancaster D, Pearson A, Flux GD. Dosimetry for fractionated (131)I-mIBG therapies in patients with primary resistant high-risk neuroblastoma: preliminary results. Cancer Biother Radiopharm. 2007;22:105–12.

104. Bodey RK, Flux GD, Evans PM. Combining dosimetry for targeted radionuclide and external beam therapies using the biologically effective dose. Cancer Biother Radiopharm. 2003;18:89–97.

105. Koral KF, Wang XH, Sisson JC, Botti J, Meyer L, Mallette S, Glazer GM, Adler RS. Calculating radiation absorbed dose for pheochromocytoma tumors in 131-I MIBG therapy. Int J Radiat Oncol Biol Phys. 1989;17:211–8.

106. Koral KF, Huberty JP, Frame B, Matthay KK, Maris JM, Regan D, Normolle D, Yanik GA. Hepatic absorbed radiation dosimetry during I-131 metaiodobenzylguanidine (MIBG) therapy for refractory neuroblastoma. Eur J Nucl Med Mol Imaging. 2008;35:2105–12.

Radiometabolic Therapy of Bone Metastases

6

Gaetano Paone and Egbert U. Nitzsche

6.1 Radiometabolic Therapy of Bone Metastases— Targeted Alpha-Particle

6.1.1 Basis of Alpha Emitter Treatment

Systemic targeted alpha-particle (α-particle) therapy represents an in-development approach of targeted radionuclide therapy for specific cancer diseases. A radionuclide is used, which undergoes alpha-decay in order to treat cancer lesions at close proximity. For example, cancer lesions originating from bony metastatic disease of castration-resistant prostatic cancer, glioma, leukemia, lymphoma, melanoma, metastatic prostate cancer presenting with lymph node and visceral metastases in addition to multiple osseous metastases, and peritoneal carcinomatosis underwent α-particle therapy [1, 2]. The primary advantage of α-particle emitters compared to β-emitting radionuclides is their very high linear energy transfer (80 keV/μm), which leads to cyto-toxic effects that are independent of the oxygen concentration, and the relative biological effectiveness. Alpha-particles deposit their energy in 70–100 μm long tracks (less than 10 cell diameters) with limited damage to the surrounding normal tissue [3]. Another important advantage is that α-particles are more likely than other types of radiation to cause double-strand breaks to DNA molecules, which is one of several effective causes of cell death. However, α-emitters are more toxic towards single cells compared to β-emitters and whether there exists a relationship between a larger skeletal tumor burden and the efficacy of Ra-223 remains to be clarified. Because of the short range of action, with its inherent overall low hematological toxicity, it is not clear, whether α-particles reach the inner marrow areas, where frequently prostate cancer cells are detected, or the inner part of larger metastases. In addition, the tumor microenvironment, especially the relation between prostate cancer cells and bone environment, needs more established insight information.

Radium-223 (Ra-223) dichloride (Xofigo®) is the first targeted systemic α-emitter therapy approach used for targeted α-particle therapy of bone metastases in patients suffering from castration-resistant prostate cancer. Ra-223 is an isotope of radium with an 11.4-day half-life. Ra-223 mimics calcium and forms complexes with the bone mineral hydroxyapatite at areas of increased bone turnover, such as bone metastases. Following intravenous injection, Xofigo® is rapidly cleared from the blood and distributed

G. Paone (✉)
Department of Nuclear Medicine and PET/CT Centre, Oncology Institute of Southern Switzerland, Bellinzona, Switzerland
e-mail: gaetano.paone@eoc.ch

E. U. Nitzsche
Department Nuclear Medicine and Molecular Imaging, Aarau General Cantonal Hospital, Aarau, Switzerland
e-mail: egbert.nitzsche@ksa.ch

© Springer Nature Switzerland AG 2019
L. Giovanella (ed.), *Nuclear Medicine Therapy*, https://doi.org/10.1007/978-3-030-17494-1_6

primarily into bone. Xofigo® is mainly eliminated by fecal excretion, while renal elimination remained very small (range 1–5%) [4, 5]. Slower intestinal transit time could potentially cause higher intestinal radiation exposure, which in turn may result in increased gastrointestinal toxicity. However, Xofigo® is not metabolized. Therefore, hepatic as well as renal function impairment is not expected to affect its pharmacokinetics. Regarding cardiac electrophysiology, no large changes in the mean QTc interval (i.e., greater than 20 ms) were detected for the calcium mimic Ra-223 up to 6 h post-dose application.

6.1.2 Indications, Contraindications, and Practical Remarks for Xofigo® Therapy of Bony Metastatic Disease in Patients Presenting with Castration-Resistant Prostate Cancer

Xofigo® is indicated as a single agent therapy for the treatment of castration-resistant prostate cancer (CRPC) with symptomatic skeletal metastases and no known visceral metastatic disease. It is approved for a course of 6 cycles.

The use of additional cycles and combinatorial strategies is currently evaluated in ongoing studies. Several guidelines assigned a level 1 evidence to Xofigo® for use in CRPC patients with bone metastases who did or did not receive taxane-based chemotherapy, for example, the American Society of Oncology, European Society for Medical Oncology, European Association of Urology, and American Urological Association, whereas the NCCN guidelines recommend Xofigo® after use of the first novel hormone. As greater insights into specific biomarkers, such as somatic or germline mutations targeted by poly ADP ribose polymerase (PARP) inhibitors develop, Xofigo® is of potential interest too. Xofigo® may prove beneficial in patients with splice variant, such as androgen-receptor splice variant 7 messenger RNA (AR-V7), that might render novel oral hormonal agents less advantageous.

Since multimodality therapy, e.g., the right therapeutic for the right patient at the right time for individualized cancer therapy is progressing, optimal timing is important. Five substances with three different mechanisms of action are currently available for the treatment of mCRPC patients (Table 6.1). All of them have demonstrated a statistically significant survival benefit in randomized phase 3 trials: The two chemotherapeutic drugs docetaxel and cabazitaxel, the α-radiator Xofigo® and the androgen receptor signaling pathway inhibitors abiraterone and enzalutamide [6–12]. The ultimate place for the use of Xofigo® is unclear. However, the use of Xofigo® as the last treatment option has not proved successful. Studies are currently investigating the use in first-line therapy in combination with abiraterone or enzalutamide, and initial results are expected by the end of 2018. The right time window enables:

– The opportunity to administer all 6 cycles within an individual multimodal therapy regimen of choice.

Regarding the opportunity to administer all 6 cycles of Xofigo®, a recent study investigated the previous and concurrent mCRPC therapies and laboratory data that are associated with the number of Xofigo® doses received. The investigators obtained the following results: Twenty-five patients (18.5%) received 1–2 radium-223 doses, 27 (20.0%) received 3–4, and 83 (61.5%) received 5–6. The most common reasons for treatment discontinuation included disease progression (61.5%, $n = 40$), patient preference (15.4%, $n = 10$), and toxicity (10.8%, $n = 7$). Factors associated with therapy completion in univariate analysis included previous sipuleucel-T treatment ($P = 0.068$), no previous abiraterone or enzalutamide treatment ($P = 0.007$), hemoglobin ≥ lower limit of normal (LLN; $P = 0.006$), white blood cell count ≥ LLN ($P = 0.045$), absolute neutrophil count (ANC) ≥ LLN ($P = 0.049$), lower alkaline phosphatase ($P = 0.029$), and lower lactate dehydrogenase levels ($P = 0.014$). Factors associated with therapy completion in multivariable analysis included previous sipuleucel-T treatment ($P = 0.009$), hemoglobin ≥ LLN ($P = 0.037$), and ANC ≥ LLN ($P = 0.029$). Therefore, it appears that several clinical parameters are associated with Xofigo® therapy completion. Overall, these

Table 6.1 Flowchart to choose a first-line treatment in CRPC with symptomatic bone metastases, no visceral lesion

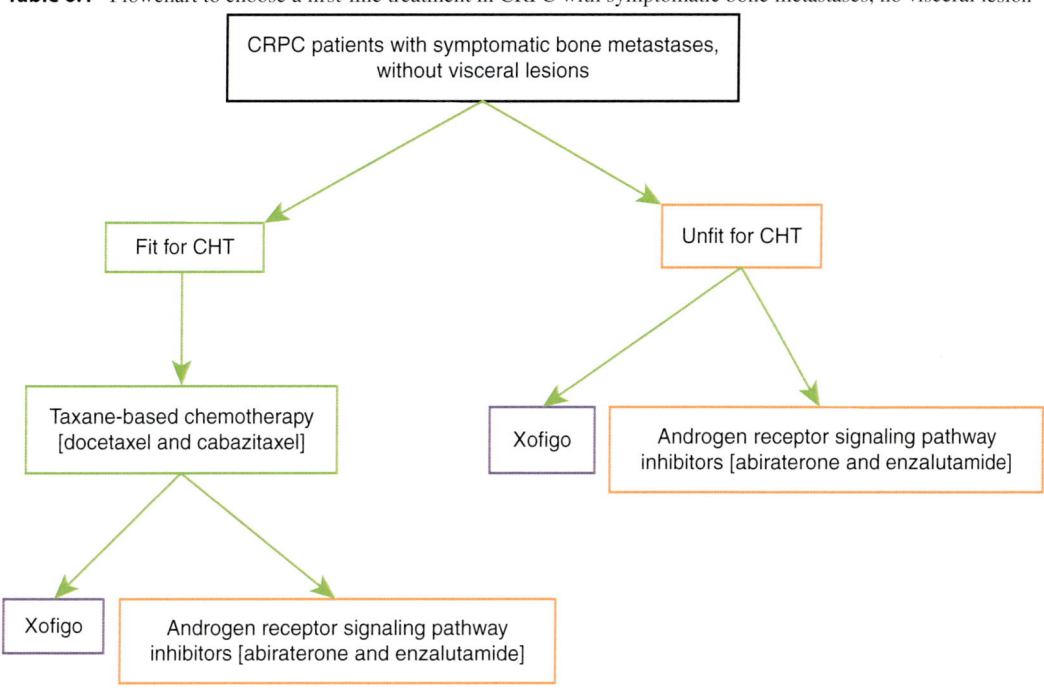

parameters potentially reflect earlier disease stage and require prospective testing [13].

A recent multivariate analyses of data from ALSYMPCA trial patients carried out by Vogelzang et al. [14] identified baseline factors that may increase hematologic toxicity risk with Xofigo® such as extent of disease and degree of prostate-specific antigen elevation, which were predictive of grade 2–4 anemia; prior docetaxel, and decreased hemoglobin and platelets, both were predictive of grade 2–4 thrombocytopenia. Patients with these factors require close monitoring during Xofigo® therapy. Further, grade 3/4 thrombocytopenia was more common in Xofigo® versus placebo patients (6% vs. 2%). Logistic regression analyses identified significant baseline predictors for grade 2–4 hematologic toxicities related to Xofigo® treatment: extent of disease (6–20 vs. < 6 bone metastases; odds ratio [OR] = 2.76; $P = 0.022$) and elevated prostate-specific antigen (OR = 1.65; $P = 0.006$) for anemia; prior docetaxel (OR = 2.16; $P = 0.035$), decreased hemoglobin (OR = 1.35; $P = 0.008$), and decreased platelets (OR = 1.44; $P = 0.030$) for thrombocytopenia. Neutropenia events were too few in placebo patients for a comparative

analysis. There were no significant associations between hematologic toxicities and number of Xofigo® injections received (4–6 vs. 1–3). This means that hematotoxicity is not cumulative.

Of note, blood count follow-up of erythrocytes at least over the last 3 months without continuous decrease, which signalizes probable early discontinuation of Xofigo® therapy, is important in order to enable the patient to receive most likely all six treatment cycles. Moreover, in that way the major goals of Xofigo® treatment, e.g., prolongation of overall survival, delay of skeletal-related adverse events, pain relief, and subsequently improvement of the quality of life may be achieved best.

However, some current contraindications such as jaw osteonecrosis, spinal cord compression, recent fractures, and inflammatory bowel disease (for example, Crohn's disease and ulcerative colitis) may be specifically investigated in the future.

Data about pain should be collected based on a structured interview: Pain localization and score (based on a visual analog pain scale), number and type of analgetic treatment. The bone metastasis osteoblastic activity must be confirmed by functional bone imaging [bone scan

(Figs. 6.1 and 6.2) or sodium fluoride positron emission tomography/computed tomography].

Before starting the Xofigo® treatment, patients need to have platelet count ≥100*10⁹/L, hemoglobin level ≥ 10 g/dL, and absolute neutrophil count ≥1.5*10⁹/L. Patients can undergo Xofigo® treatment and follow-up as outpatients, because the estimated radiation dose to caregivers and household members is very low, 2 μSv h − 1 MBq − 1 on contact and 0.02 μSv h − 1 MBq − 1 at 1 m immediately after administration [15].

6.1.3 Results of Xofigo® Therapy of Bony Metastatic Disease in Patients Presenting with Castration-Resistant Prostate Cancer

6.1.3.1 Overall Survival

Based on the ALSYMPCA trial, Xofigo® proved effective regarding the improvement of overall survival [14.9 months vs. 11.3 months; hazard ratio (HR) = 0.70, 95% confidence interval (CI) = 0.58−0.83; p = 0.00185)] [7].

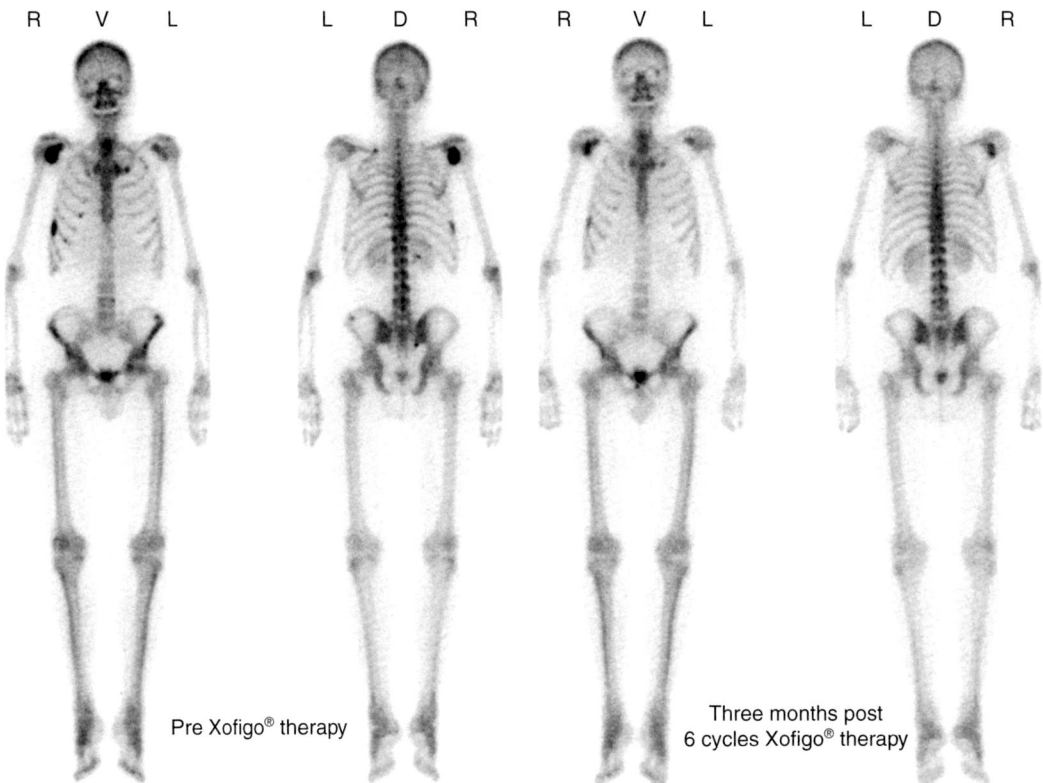

Pre Xofigo® therapy

Three months post
6 cycles Xofigo® therapy

Fig. 6.1 Bone scan response in a 55-year-old patient presenting with castration-resistant metastatic prostate cancer and multiple bone metastases prior to Xofigo® therapy and regressed metastatic bone disease 3 months after completion of six therapy cycles. Legend: There are multiple findings of increased osteoblastic activity representing metastatic spread of prostate cancer into the skeleton within the scapula, ribs, and pelvis bilaterally as well as the vertebral column, while the follow-up bone scan three months after completion of Xofigo® therapy demonstrates markedly reduced osteoblastic activity in the reference lesions of the right scapula, vertebra TH 6, and ribs 6/7 right anterolateral, whereas multiple smaller lesions within the ribs and pelvic skeleton disappeared

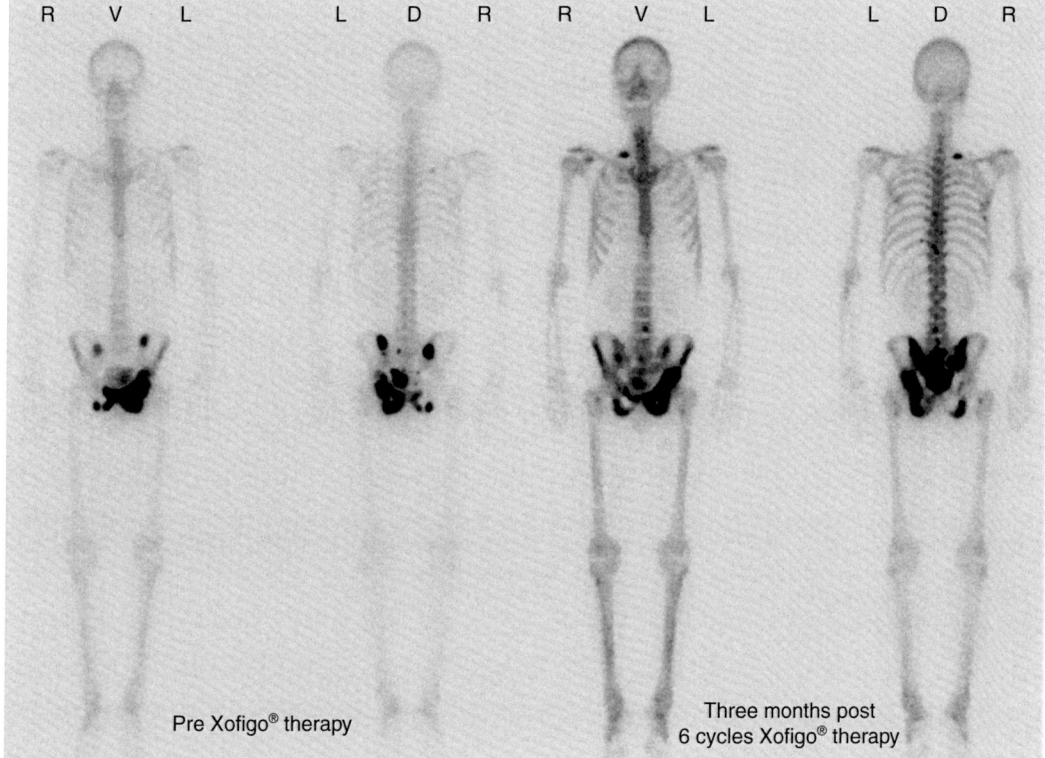

Fig. 6.2 Bone scan representing progressive bony metastatic disease in a 62-year-old patient presenting with castration-resistant metastatic prostate cancer and multiple bone metastases prior to Xofigo® therapy and progressive disease 3 months after completion of six therapy cycles. Legend: There are multiple findings of increased osteoblastic activity representing metastatic spread of prostate cancer into the skeleton within the pelvis bilaterally as well as one rib lesion in the fourth rib dorsal right sided. Three months after completion of Xofigo® therapy the follow-up bone scan demonstrates despite the known metastatic lesion in the pelvic bone new metastatic bone lesions outside the pelvic skeleton representing progressive bony metastatic disease

6.1.3.2 Delay of Skeletal-Related Adverse Events

The time until the onset of skeletal events was prolonged (15.6 vs. 9.8 months; HR = 0.66, 95% CI = 0.52−0.83; $p < 0.001$) [16].

6.1.3.3 Improvement of the Quality of Life

The quality of life was improved ($p = 0.02$) and deterioration in ECOG-PS of two or more points was significantly lower in the Xofigo® treated group (HR = 0.62, 95% CI = 0.46−0.85; $p = 0.003$). In addition, healthcare resource use (HCRU), including hospitalization events and days, were prospectively collected in the ALSYMPCA trial. Subsequently healthcare resource use for the first 12 months post-randomization was investigated. Significantly fewer Xofigo® (218/589; 37.0%) vs. placebo patients (133/292; 45.5%) had at least one hospitalization event ($P = 0.016$). However, mean number of hospitalization events per patient was similar (Xofigo® 0.69 vs. placebo 0.79, $P = 0.226$), likely due to the significantly longer follow-up time for Xofigo® (7.82 months vs. 6.92 months for placebo) [17].

6.1.3.4 Treatment Monitoring

Regularly, six Xofigo® iv injections are given in 4-week treatment intervals over six months. Whenever possible, the Xofigo® treatment should be a tandem care provided by (uro)oncology/nuclear medicine physicians according to the multiple eyes watching principle in an optimized therapeutic setting. Standard hematologic blood tests prior to each treatment with Xofigo® are mandatory as well as proper restaging of disease prior to initiation of Xofigo® therapy.

Circulating biomarkers like alkaline phosphatase (ALP) and prostate-specific antigen (PSA) are indicators of overall response. Unfortunately, both are indirect markers and do not provide information about individual sites of involvement. Therefore, laboratory measurement of ALP and PSA is regularly recommended prior to and 3 months after completion of Xofigo® treatment. In case of a clinical worsening of the patient with suspected progressive tumor disease or recurrence of symptoms, especially on the skeleton, an intermediate check should be performed using available on-site morphological and functional imaging approaches (evaluation of skeletal metastases, new and/or progressive lymph node metastases, new-onset of visceral metastases) and supplementary ALP and PSA check.

6.1.4 Methodology of the Treatment

European expert recommendations sharing best practice and experience to optimize Xofigo® treatment service provision and improvement of patient care have been published recently by Du Y and coworkers [18]. Key points such as:

- center organization, preparation including staff training and patient referral,
- Xofigo® ordering, preparation, and disposal,
- Xofigo® treatment delivery including initial consultation, required blood tests, and administration of the agent with a suggestion for follow-up consultation, and finally
- patient experience with regard to comfort, satisfaction, and proper information are explained.

6.1.5 Risks and Complications of the Procedure, Side Effects (Immediate/Long-Term)

6.1.5.1 Safety and Side Effects

The safety for Xofigo® therapy was demonstrated, since grade 3 and 4 myelotoxicity were infrequent [19, 20]. Nadir of myelotoxicity occurred at 2–4 weeks after treatment and recovery was observed within 24 weeks [21]. In any case, myelosuppression was dose-related and reversible. However, more common no-hematological toxicities, such as diarrhea, nausea, vomiting, and fatigue, were more frequent than with other novel therapies, such as abiraterone and enzalutamide, although easily manageable [22].

6.1.5.2 Xofigo® Re-Treatment

As indicated from initial results published recently, Xofigo® re-treatment was well tolerated in a highly selected population, with minimal hematologic toxicity, and provided continued control of disease progression in bone [23].

6.1.5.3 Carcinogenesis, Mutagenesis, Impairment of Fertility

Animal studies have not been conducted to evaluate the carcinogenic potential of Radium-223 dichloride. However, in repeat-dose toxicity studies in rats, osteosarcomas, a known effect of bone-seeking radionuclides, were observed at clinically relevant doses 7–12 months after the start of treatment. The presence of other neoplastic changes, including lymphoma and mammary gland carcinoma, was also reported in 12- to 15-month repeat-dose toxicity studies in rats.

Genetic toxicology studies have not been conducted with Radium-223 dichloride. However, the mechanism of action of Xofigo® treatment involves induction of double-strand DNA breaks, which is a known and in this case desired effect of radiation.

Animal studies have not been conducted to evaluate the effects of Xofigo® treatment on male or female fertility or reproductive function. Xofigo® may impair fertility and reproductive function in humans based on its mechanism of action.

The safety and efficacy of concomitant chemotherapy with Xofigo® have not been established. Outside of a clinical trial, concomitant use with chemotherapy is not recommended due to the potential for additive myelosuppression. If chemotherapy, other systemic radioisotopes, or hemibody external radiotherapy is administered during the treatment period, Xofigo® should be discontinued. This also applies to ongoing cortisone therapy due to the risk of bone fracture.

6.1.5.4 Secondary Malignant Neoplasms

Xofigo® contributes to a patient's overall long-term cumulative radiation exposure. Long-term cumulative radiation exposure may be associated with an increased risk of cancer and hereditary defects. Due to its mechanism of action and neoplastic changes, including osteosarcomas in rats, Xofigo® may increase the risk of osteosarcoma or other secondary malignant neoplasms. However, the overall incidence of new malignancies in the randomized trial was lower on the Xofigo® arm compared to placebo (<1% vs. 2%; respectively). The expected latency period for the development of secondary malignancies exceeded the duration of follow-up for patients in the trial. Moreover, a recent updated final long-term safety follow-up ALSYMPCA analysis shows that Xofigo® is well tolerated in CRPC patients with symptomatic bone metastases, with minimal nonhematologic adverse events, a low incidence of myelosuppression with long-term preservation of hematopoietic function, and no new safety issues [24].

6.1.5.5 Interactions with Other Drugs Concurrently Used

Subgroup analyses indicated that the concurrent use of bisphosphonates or calcium channel blockers did not affect the safety and efficacy of Xofigo® in the randomized clinical trial. Regardless of baseline opioid use, a favorable safety profile in castration-resistant prostate cancer patients with symptomatic bone metastases was observed [25].

6.1.6 Summary

To date it is established that Xofigo® improves survival and the quality of life in patients suffering from castration-resistant prostate cancer with symptomatic bone metastases. It prolongs the time until the onset of skeletal events. The safety for Xofigo® therapy was demonstrated, since grade 3 and 4 myelotoxicity were infre-

quent. Six Xofigo® iv injections are given in 4-week treatment intervals over six months. Whenever possible, the Xofigo® treatment should be a tandem care provided by (uro) oncology/nuclear medicine physicians according to the multiple eyes watching principle in an optimized therapeutic setting. Standard blood tests prior to each treatment with Xofigo® are mandatory as well as proper restaging of disease prior to initiation of Xofigo® therapy. The right time window (yet to be defined more precisely) enables the opportunity to administer all 6 cycles within an individual multimodal therapy regimen (Table 6.2).

In the future Xofigo® may not be administered in castration-resistant prostate cancer patients with symptomatic bone metastases only, but also in patients presenting with metastatic high-risk osteosarcoma and metastatic bone disease in hormone-refractory breast cancer as indicated from ongoing trials [26, 27].

Table 6.2 Xofigo quick use-guide

Indication	CRPC with symptomatic skeletal metastases and no known visceral metastatic disease
Administration	Six Xofigo® iv injections are given in 4-week treatment intervals over 6 months
Blood test pre-therapy	Plt count $\geq 100*10^9$/L, Hb level ≥ 10 g/dL, ANC count $\geq 1.5*10^9$/L.
Treatment monitoring	Standard blood tests prior to each treatment are mandatory
Hematological side effect	Grade 3/4 myelotoxicity (Infrequent). Nadir at 2–4 weeks after treatment and recovery within 24 weeks.
Non-hematological side effect	Diarrhea, nausea, vomiting, and fatigue
Concomitant therapy	Concomitant chemotherapy or EBRT with Xofigo® have not been established and is not recommended. If chemotherapy, other systemic radioisotopes or hemibody external radiotherapy are administered during the treatment period, Xofigo® should be discontinued
Interactions with other drugs	Concurrent use of bisphosphonates or calcium channel blockers did not affect the safety and efficacy of Xofigo®

6.2 Radiometabolic Therapy of Bone Metastases—Targeted Beta-Particle

6.2.1 Basis of Beta Emitter Treatment

Radionuclide therapy with beta-particle (β-particle) plays a crucial role in the palliative regimen of metastatic bone pain, representing a valid alternative and support in the drugs sequence to treat cancer-induced bone pain. The ideal radionuclide for the treatment of bone metastases presents the following characteristics: selective uptake by bone metastases, rapid clearance from soft tissues and healthy bone, energy emission between 0.8 and 2 MeV, bio-distribution similar to that of diphosphonates, limited irradiation of the bone marrow, prompt availability, and reasonable costs [28–30].

Beta-emitting radionuclides, compared to α-particles, deposit their energy in 50–10.000 μm long tracks with relative limited damage to the surrounding normal tissue causing a single-strand breaks to DNA molecules, generally easy to repair with less likely to introduce cellular death. As previously described these radionuclides exploiting their high LET (even if lower than the α-particles, Table 6.3) directly on the neoplastic cells (magic bullet), regulating in particular the surrounding inflammatory reaction, thus temporarily reducing the pain, with a modest amount of side effects. The therapeutic effect is mainly due to a lower release of pain modulatory agents, as cytokines and interferon, from tumor microenvironment, reduced activation of periosteum nociceptors, edema and inflammatory reaction with associated decrease of interstitial pressure and algogenic substances release. These bone-seeking radiopharmaceuticals have a specific affinity for bone remodeling sites and are classified as osteotropic drug [31–34].

Multiple β-emitting radionuclides had been evaluated and used clinically prior to the development of radium-223 (Table 6.4). The most widely studied are strontium-89 (89-Sr), samarium-153 (153-Sm), Phosphorus-32, and Rhenium-186. In clinical application the most widely used are: 89-Sr (Metastron), 153-Sm EDTMP (Quadramet). 89-Sr is an alkaline-earth metal, belongs to the same periodic family as calcium, able to bind to the bone without a carrier. It is marketed as chloride ($89SrCl2$), rapidly eliminated by urinary tract while 50% of the administered dose binds bone structure. 153Sm-EDTMP is a chelated complex of a radioisotope (Samarium with EDTMP) that exhibits similar binding properties to the diphosphonates used for bone scintigraphy. It is rapidly removed from the bloodstream with the urine and has a binding of 60% of the administered dose [35–37].

6.2.2 Indications, Contraindications, and Practical Remarks for Beta-Emitters Therapy of Bony Metastatic Disease

Radiometabolic therapy with β-emitters is a targeted and selective treatment of metastatic bone localizations and is performed for analgesic purposes. Further indication could be primary

Table 6.4 Radionuclide (β-emitters) characteristics

Radionuclide	T ½ (d)	Eβ(MeV) med/max	Range (mm) max	Dose (mCi)
89-Sr (SrCl²)	50.5	0.58/1.46	6.8	4
153-Sm (EDTMP)	1.9	0.35/0.80	3.3	0.5–1/ Kg
32-P (Phosphate)	14.2	0.69/1.7	8.0	3–12
186-Re (HEDP)	3.7	0.36/1.07	4.7	25–35

Table 6.3 Comparison of absorbed doses for red bone marrow and bone surface for selected osteotropic radiotherapeutics

	89-Sr	153-Sm	223-Ra
Radiation	Beta	Beta	Alpha
Administered dose (MBq)	148	2590	21
Absorbed dose rBm (Gy)	1.628	3.988	1.50
Absorbed dose BSF (Gy)	2.516	17.508	16

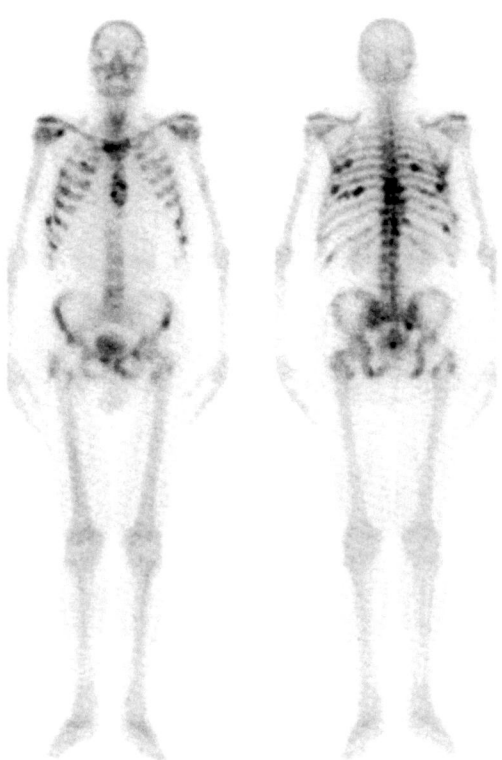

Fig. 6.3 Bone scan evaluation pre-radionuclide therapy with 153-Sm in a 66-year-old patient presenting with CRPC. Legend: Positive bone scan with multiple findings of increased osteoblastic activity representing metastatic spread of prostate cancer into the skeleton in patient with diffuse bone pain

ity of life, performance status, estimated life expectancy, patient compliance) and generally require a stepwise approach to pain management led by variety of therapeutic options available. Chemotherapy, targeted therapies, and hormone therapy may contribute to pain relief by reducing tumor bulk and/or by modulating pain-signaling pathways. In the late stage of disease few drugs are effective, making necessary other therapeutic approach as radiation therapy and recently bisphosphonate in addition to the analgesic strategy. Bone-targeted radionuclide therapy, for its effectiveness and safety profile, fits into this scenario as a valid option for pain palliation in diffuse bony disease and are generally reserved for individuals with persistent or recurrent multifocal bone pain after EBRT and/or other forms of therapy. Generally 153-Sm is approved for pain palliation in patients with confirmed osteoblastic bone lesions that enhance on radionuclide bone scan, while 89-Sr is approved for the relief of bone pain in patients with painful skeletal metastases [39].

painful bone tumors when confirmed by areas of intense uptake on bone scintigraphy; however, this indication is not yet approved.

Prerequisite for bone-targeted radionuclide treatment is a positive bone scan and associated diffuse bone pain (Fig. 6.3). Contextual general condition are: refractory bone pain to minor analgesic therapy or opioid therapy in increasing doses, life expectancy >3 months, no cytotoxic chemotherapy and/or radiation therapy a few weeks (6 weeks) prior to treatment and preserved bone marrow reserve (BCC: Hb > 90 g/L; WCC > 3.5 × 10^9/L, PLT > 100 × 10^9/L) and renal function (Creatinine 0.5–1.5 mg/mL) [38].

The most appropriate treatment choice may be complex, influenced by multiple factors (qual-

6.2.2.1 Contraindications of Bone-Targeted Radiopharmaceutical Therapy

Absolute contraindications are: pregnancy, breastfeeding, acute or chronic renal failure (creatinine >1.8 mg/mL and or glomerular filtration rate < 30 mL/min), acute spinal cord compression and myelosuppression (PLT < 60 × 10^9, leukocytes less than 2.5 × 10^9/L), a life expectancy <1 month.

Relative contraindications are: predominant extra-skeletal metastatic involvement, diffuse medullary involvement defined as "superscan" on bone scintigraphy (Fig. 6.4) with higher risk of myelotoxicity, chemotherapy and/or radiotherapy performed in the previous 6 weeks, disseminated intravascular coagulation (DIC) with associated risk factor for severe thrombocytopenia, myelosuppression (PLT < 100 × 10^9/L), pathological fracture (therapy feasible only in association with prosthesis and/or external RT and evidence of other metastatic sites) [40, 41].

6.2.3 Results of Beta-Emitters Therapy of Bony Metastatic Disease

The main objectives in the management of patient with bone metastases are: optimization of pain control, preservation and restoration of function, stabilization of the skeleton, reduction of risk of skeletal-related events (SRE), quality of life and improvement of local tumor control. The widespread and constant bone pain remains the most disabling symptom and is not easily managed.

6.2.3.1 Pain Palliation

Bone-targeted radioisotope therapy offers a beneficial effect on pain control in patients with osteoblastic or mixed pattern (osteoblastic/osteoclastic) metastases [33, 34].

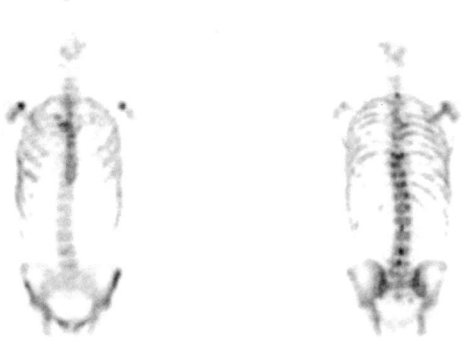

R ANT L   L POST R

Fig. 6.4 Bone scan evaluation in a 73-year-old patient presenting with CRPC. diffuse medullary involvement defined as "superscan" on bone scintigraphy. Legend: Positive bone scan with diffuse medullary involvement defined as "superscan" and considered as relative contraindication for radionuclide therapy with β-emitters

The main advantage is represented by rapidly, selectively, and simultaneously targeting of all bone lesions.

Several clinical trials confirm that β-emitters can achieve bone pain relief with response rate between 50 and 95%, including a complete relief in about 15–30% of patients [42–44]. Single treatment can achieve pain relief in about 70% of patient for 89-Sr and 153-Sm, otherwise combination with other therapies is slightly more effective with pain palliation in 74% of patients with prostate or breast cancer [45].

153-Sm was compared with placebo in two randomized phase III trials. Both found that treatment with β-emitter was more effective than placebo in providing pain relief [46, 47].

The effects of bone-targeted radiopharmaceutical therapy in breast cancer was underlined in a systematic review that confirm a moderate bone pain palliation with low evidence in terms of supporting the clinical effect in relieving pain [48].

Pain palliation has a latency period from the administration time taking up to one to four weeks and that is usually shorter for the 153-Sm than 89-Sr. The palliative effect lasts 2–4 months after the administration of the 153-Sm and from 3 to 6 months after administration of 89-Sr (Table 6.5). Generally lithic bone metastases showed a worse response (42%) than osteoblastic (62.50%) or mixed pattern (60%) [49, 50].

6.2.3.2 Quality of Life and Survival

Radionuclide treatment proved effective regarding the improvement of quality of life in patients with osteoblastic or mixed pattern metastases [51, 52].

Few results highlighted survival benefits after radionuclide therapy with β-emitters, particularly a phase II study in prostate cancer showed a survival benefit if chemotherapy was added to 89-Sr (27.7 vs. 16.8 months) [53].

6.2.3.3 Combination of Radionuclide Therapy and Other Treatments

Bone-targeted radionuclide therapy, in patients with multiple sites of symptomatic bone metastases, offers a similar degree of pain relief than external hemi-body radiation and may be asso-

Table 6.5 Effect on pain palliation and myelotoxicity of β-emitters

Radionuclide	% reduction pain	% complete relief	Duration (m)	Latency (w)	Myelotoxicity
89-Sr	50–75	15–30	3–6	<2 w	Moderate
153-Sm	65–75	30	2–4	1–3 w	Low

ciated with less myelotoxicity. External beam radiotherapy (EBRT) represents the treatment of choice if the bone scan is negative and in cases of imminent pathological fracture. Combination of EBRT and radionuclide therapy should be evaluated only in selected patients [54].

No evidence-based data support concomitant or sequential use of radionuclide therapy and chemotherapy due to the possible myelotoxicity. Normally it is preferable to avoid long-acting myelosuppressive chemotherapy 4–6 weeks prior to the β-emitter administration. After bone-seeking radionuclide treatment (indifferently 89-Sr, 153-Sm), systemic chemotherapy should be avoided for about 12 weeks. Among the few data reported in literature certainly the TRAPEZE trial reports interesting result, in a cohort of 757 patients, suggesting improved clinical progression-free survival after 89-Sr combined with docetaxel without evident benefits in terms of OS and SRE free-interval [55].

Different studies support, instead, concomitant or sequential use of radionuclide therapy and bisphosphonates despite previous data underlined the possible reduced uptake of bone-target radionuclide. In particular, recent studies indicate absence of competition between bisphosphonates and 153-Sm or 89-Sr [56–58].

6.2.4 Methodology of the Treatment

EANM guideline published recently by Handkiewicz-Junak et al. shared best practice and experience to optimize radionuclide treatment in patient with bone metastases suggesting, whenever possible, a multidisciplinary approach provided by nuclear medicine physician, a medical oncologist, and a radiation oncologist according to the multiple eyes watching principle in an optimized therapeutic setting.

Mandatory procedures to be performed before treatment are: medical history, life expectancy estimation, radiological imaging, bone scan, complete blood count, renal function evaluation, and pregnancy test. In the absence of contraindication, there are not specific patient preparation to implement before the treatment. Patients should be informed about the risk of a possible initial increase in bone pain (pain flare phenomenon) and that its reduction occurs within 2–4 weeks after therapy.

Center organization, trained and certified staff, radionuclide ordering, preparation, and disposal are key points to administer radionuclide therapy.

Bone-seeking radionuclide should be administered intravenously slowly over 1–2 min, using appropriate precautions for handling and disposal, followed by 0.9% saline flush. If extravasation occurs it is necessary to stop infusion. It is mandatory to measure with a properly calibrated active meter radio-drug activity. Generally recommended doses are 37 MBq/Kg for 153-Sm and 150 MBq (4 millicurie [mCi] or 1.5–2.2 MBq/Kg) for 89-Sr. (Table 6.4).

Re-treatment, in case of pain recurrence, should be based on individual response, symptoms, and blood counts and are generally not recommended at intervals <90 days (10–12 weeks for 153-Sm and 12 weeks for 89-Sr) [38, 59, 60].

6.2.5 Risks and Complications of the Procedure, Side Effects (Immediate/Long-Term)

Adverse reactions are very rare and frequency not defined. A flushing sensation has been reported following rapid (<30 s) injection. No suspected/dangerous interactions with other drug were found.

6.2.5.1 Immediate Side Effects

Pain-flair phenomenon is a transient increase in bone-pain. It usually occurs in about 5–15% of cases and generally within 72 h after administration. This symptom is temporary and responding to a common analgesic therapy. It represents an "inflammatory" reaction caused by irradiation and is considered a positive-response indicator to the treatment associated with a good clinical response.

Nausea and vomiting are very rare, particularly observed in patients with diffuse bone involvement [39, 61].

6.2.5.2 Long-Term Side Effects

Frequent moderate transient myelotoxicity is observed, predominantly affecting thrombocyte and leukocyte. Nadir and recovery times are usually related to the individual condition and radioactivity. Generally bone marrow depression begins after 2 weeks, nadir at 3–5 weeks (153 Sm) or 12–16 weeks (89-Sr) with complete or partial recovery within 3–6 months.

Myelosuppression with grade 3 or 4 toxicity is strictly related to previous therapy, bone marrow reserve and may be exacerbated by bone marrow replacement in case of extensive bone involvement. Use is not recommended in patients with severely impaired bone marrow function by prior therapies or diffuse disease infiltration (unless potential benefit outweighs risks).

Monitor blood-count may be useful for up to 6 weeks after treatment with 153-Sm. After 89-Sr administration longer follow-up is required because of prolonged and more evident myelotoxicity (12–16 weeks) [38, 62].

6.2.5.3 Radiation Safety Procedure

Pregnancy should be avoided for at least 6–8 months following treatment. In case of treatment on an outpatient basis, patients remain in the nuclear medicine department for 4–6 h after administration to assess any early side effects. Particular precaution is necessary for urinary radiopharmaceutical excretion during the first 24–48 h after injection. Patients must comply rigorous hygiene rules to avoid contamination using the same toilet facility. Inpatient treatment required rigorous radiation safety instructions for nursing personnel; urinary catheterization is necessary for incontinent patients (to minimize radioactive contamination of clothing, bedding, and/or environment) [38, 39].

6.2.6 Summary

Radionuclide therapy with β-emitters is purely palliative in case of symptomatic bone metastases refractory to analgesics/opioid therapy. Key clinical aspects are life expectancy superior >3 months, no cytotoxic chemotherapy and/or radiation therapy a few weeks (6 weeks) prior to treatment and conserved bone marrow reserve (Table 6.6). To date it is established that bone-targeted radionuclide therapy offers a beneficial effect on pain control and improvement of quality of life in patients with osteoblastic or mixed pattern (osteoblastic/osteoclastic) metastases. The main advantage is represented by rapidly, selectively, and simultaneously targeting of all bone lesions. No evident data were highlighted in terms of survival and concomitant or sequential use of β-emitters therapy with EBRT and chemotherapy. Contrarily the concomitant/sequential use with bisphosphonates is indicate in clinical routine. Life expectancy estimation, bone scan and radiological imaging, complete blood count, renal function evaluation, pregnancy test are mandatory prior to initiation of therapy. The safety was demonstrated with moderate myelotoxicity, exacerbated by bone marrow replacement in case of extensive bone involvement. Use is not recommended in patients with severely impaired bone marrow function by prior therapies or diffuse bone infiltration. Monitor blood-count is useful after treatment (for up to 6 weeks with 153-Sm and 12–16 weeks after 89-Sr).

Table 6.6 β-Emitters quick use-guide

Indication	Palliative treatment in symptomatic bony metastatic disease refractory to analgesics/opioid therapy
Administration	β-emitters radionuclide should be administered intravenously slowly over 1–2 min
Blood test pre-therapy	Hb > 90 g/L; WCC > 3.5 × 10⁹/L, PLT > 100 × 10⁹/L
Re-treatment	Based on individual response, symptoms, blood counts and generally not recommended at intervals <90 days
Hematological side effect	Transient myelotoxicity predominantly affecting thrombocyte and leukocyte. Nadir at 3–5 weeks (153 Sm) or 12–16 weeks (89-Sr) with complete or partial recovery within 3–6 months.
Non-hematological side effect	Pain-flair phenomenon (transient increase in bone-pain). Nausea and vomiting are very rare, particularly observed in patients with diffuse bone involvement
Concomitant therapy	Combination of EBRT and radionuclide therapy should be evaluated only in selected patients. No data support concomitant or sequential use of radionuclide therapy and chemotherapy. Normally is preferable to avoid long-acting myelosuppressive chemotherapy 4–6 weeks prior to the β-emitter administration. After Bone-seeking radionuclide treatment (indifferently 89-Sr, 153-Sm), systemic chemotherapy should be avoid for about 12 weeks
Interactions with other drugs	Concomitant or sequential use of radionuclide therapy and bisphosphonates did not affect the safety and efficacy of treatments

The blood test values above contain: Hb > 90 g/L; WCC > 3.5×10^9/L, PLT > 100×10^9/L

References

1. Mulford DA, Scheinberg DA, Jurcic JG. The promise of targeted alpha-particle therapy. J Nucl Med. 2005;46(Suppl 1):199S–204S.
2. Kratochwil C, Bruchertseifer F, Rathke H, Bronzel M, Apostolidis C, Weichert W, et al. Targeted α-therapy of metastatic castration-resistant prostate cancer with 225Ac-PSMA-617: dosimetry estimate and empiric dose finding. J Nucl Med. 2017;58(10):1624–163.
3. Elgqvist J, Frost S, Pouget JP, Albertsson P. The potential and hurdles of targeted alpha therapy—clinical trials and beyond. Front Oncol. 2014;3:324.
4. Bruland OS, Larsen RH. Radium revisited. In: Bruland OS, Flagstad T, editors. Targeted cancer therapies: an odyssey. Ravnetrykk No. 29: University Library of Tromso; 2003. p. 195–202.
5. "Preparation and use of radium-223 to target calcified tissues for pain palliation, bone cancer therapy, and bone surface conditioning" US 6635234 http://patft.uspto.gov
6. Tannock IF, de Wit R, Berry WR, Horti J, Pluzanska A, Chi KN, et al. Docetaxel plus prednisone or mitoxantrone plus prednisone for advanced prostate cancer. N Engl J Med. 2004;351(15):1502–12.
7. Parker C, Nilsson S, Heinrich D, Helle SI, O'Sullivan JM, Fossa SD, et al. Alpha emitter radium-223 and survival in metastatic prostate cancer. N Engl J Med. 2013;369(3):213–23.
8. de Bono JS, Oudard S, Ozguroglu M, Hansen S, Machiels JP, Kocak I, et al. Prednisone plus cabazitaxel or mitoxantrone for metastatic castration-resistant prostate cancer progressing after docetaxel treatment: a randomised open-label trial. Lancet. 2010;376(9747):1147–54.
9. de Bono JS, Logothetis CJ, Molina A, Fizazi K, North S, Chu L, et al. Abiraterone and increased survival in metastatic prostate cancer. N Engl J Med. 2011;364(21):1995–2005.
10. Ryan CJ, Smith MR, de Bono JS, Molina A, Logothetis CJ, de Souza P, et al. Abiraterone in metastatic prostate cancer without previous chemotherapy. N Engl J Med. 2013;368(2):138–48.
11. Beer TM, Armstrong AJ, Rathkopf DE, Loriot Y, Sternberg CN, Higano CS, et al. Enzalutamide in metastatic prostate cancer before chemotherapy. N Engl J Med. 2014;371(5):424–33.
12. Scher HI, Fizazi K, Saad F, Taplin ME, Sternberg CN, Miller MD, et al. Increased survival with enzalutamide in prostate cancer after chemotherapy. N Engl J Med. 2012;367:1187–97.
13. McKay RR, Jacobus S, Fiorillo M, Ledet EM, Cotogna PM, Steinberger AE, et al. Radium-223 use in clinical practice and variables associated with completion of therapy. Clin Genitourin Cancer. 2016;15(2):e289–98.
14. Vogelzang NJ, Coleman RE, Michalski JM, Nilsson S, O'Sullivan JM, Parker C, et al. Hematologic safety of Radium-223 dichloride: baseline prognostic factors associated with myelosuppression in the ALSYMPCA trial. Clin Genitourin Cancer. 2016;15(1):42–52.
15. Dauer LT, Williamson MJ, Humm J, O'Donoghue J, Ghani R, Awadallah R, et al. Radiation safety considerations for the use of Ra-223 in men with castration-resistant prostate cancer. Health Phys. 2014;106(4):494–504.
16. Sartor O, Coleman R, Nilsson S, Heinrich D, Helle SI, O'Sullivan JM, et al. Effect of radium-223 dichloride on symptomatic skeletal events in patients with castration-resistant prostate cancer and bone metastases: results from a phase 3, double-blind, randomised trial. Lancet Oncol. 2014;15:738–46.

17. Parker C, Zhan L, Cislo P, Reuning-Scherer J, Vogelzang NJ, Nilsson S, et al. Effect of radium-223 dichloride (Ra-223) on hospitalisation: an analysis from the phase 3 randomised alpharadin in symptomatic prostate cancer patients (ALSYMPCA) trial. Eur J Cancer. 2017;71:1–6.

18. Du Y, Carrio I, De Vincentis G, Fanti S, Ilhan H, Mommsen C, et al. Practical recommendations for radium-223 treatment of metastatic castration-resistant prostate cancer. Eur J Nucl Med Mol Imaging. 2017;44(10):1671–8.

19. Nilsson S, Larsen RH, Fosså SD, Balteskard L, Borch KW, Westlin JE, et al. First clinical experience with alpha-emitting radium-223 in the treatment of skeletal metastases. Clin Cancer Res. 2005;11:4451–9.

20. Nilsson S, Franzén L, Parker C, Tyrrell C, Blom R, Tennvall J, et al. Bone-targeted radium-223 in symptomatic, hormonerefractory prostate cancer: a randomised, multicentre, placebocontrolled phase II study. Lancet Oncol. 2007;8:587–94.

21. Pandit-Taskar N, Larson SM, Carrasquillo JA. Bone-seeking radiopharmaceuticals for treatment of osseous metastases, part 1: α therapy with 223Ra-dichloride. J Nucl Med. 2014;55:268–74.

22. Vuong W, Sartor O, Pal SK. Radium-223 in metastatic castration resistant prostate cancer. Asian J Androl. 2014;16:348–53.

23. Keizman D, Nordquist LT, Mariados N, Méndez Vidal MJ, Thellenberg Karlsson C, Peer A, et al. Radium-223 (Ra-223) re-treatment (re-tx): Experience from an international, multicenter, prospective study in patients (pts) with castration-resistant prostate cancer and bone metastases (mCRPC). Eur Urol Suppl. 2016;15(3):e764.

24. Parker CC, Coleman RE, Sartor O, Vogelzang NJ, Bottomley D, Heinrich D, et al. Three-year safety of Radium-223 dichloride in patients with castration-resistant prostate cancer and symptomatic bone metastases from phase 3 randomized alpharadin in symptomatic prostate cancer trial. Eur Urol. 2017; https://doi.org/10.1016/j.eururo.2017.06.021.

25. Parker C, Finkelstein SF, Michalski JM, O'Sullivan JM, Bruland Ø, Vogelzang NJ, et al. Efficacy and safety of Radium-223 dichloride in symptomatic castration-resistant prostate cancer patients with or without baseline opioid use from the phase 3 ALSYMPCA trial. Eur Urol. 2016;70(5):875–83.

26. Subbiah V, Anderson P, Rohren E. Alpha emitter radium 223 in high-risk osteosarcoma—first clinical evidence of response and blood-brain barrier penetration. JAMA Oncol. 2015;1(2):253–5.

27. Takalkar A, Adams S, Subbiah V. Radium-223 dichloride bone-targeted alpha particle therapy for hormone-refractory breast cancer metastatic to bone. Exp Hematol Oncol. 2014;3:23.

28. Bouchet LG, Bolch WE, Goddu SM, Howell RW, Rao DV. Considerations in the selection of radiopharmaceuticals for palliation of bone pain from metastatic osseous lesions. J Nucl Med. 2000;41(4):682–7.

29. Pandit-Taskar N, Batraki M, Divgi CR. Radiopharmaceutical therapy for palliation of bone pain from osseous metastases. J Nucl Med. 2004;45(8):1358–65.

30. Hosain F, Spencer RP. Radiopharmaceuticals for palliation of metastatic osseous lesions: biologic and physical background. Semin Nucl Med. 1992;22(1):11–6.

31. Silberstein EB, Taylor AT Jr, EANM. EANM procedure guidelines for treatment of refractory metastatic bone pain. Eur J Nucl Med Mol Imaging. 2003;30(3):BP7–11.

32. Bodei L, Lam M, Chiesa C, Flux G, Brans B, Chiti A, et al. EANM procedure guideline for treatment of refractory metastatic bone pain. Eur J Nucl Med Mol Imaging. 2008;35(10):1934–40.

33. Krishnamurthy GT, Krishnamurthy S. Radionuclides for metastatic bone pain palliation: a need for rational re-evaluation in the new millennium. J Nucl Med. 2000;41:688–91.

34. Edwards GK, Santoro J, Taylor AJR. Use of bone scintigraphy to select patients with multiple myeloma for treatment with strontium-89. J Nucl Med. 1994;35:1992–3.

35. Liepe K, Kotzerke J. A comparative study of 188Re-HEDP, 186Re-HEDP, 153Sm-EDTMP and 89Sr in the treatment of painful skeletal metastases. Nucl Med Commun. 2007;28(8):623–30.

36. Liepe K, Runge R, Kotzerke J. Systemic radionuclide therapy in pain palliation. Am J Hosp Palliat Care. 2005;22(6):457–64.

37. Jong JM, Oprea-Lager DE, Hooft L, de Klerk JM, Bloemendal HJ, Verheul H, et al. Radiopharmaceuticals for palliation of bone pain in patients with castration-resistant prostate cancer metastatic to bone: a systematic review. Eur Urol. 2016;70(3):416–26.

38. Handkiewicz-Junak D, Poeppel TD, Bodei L, Aktolun C, Ezziddin S, Giammarile F, et al. EANM guidelines for radionuclide therapy of bone metastases with beta-emitting radionuclides. Eur J Nucl Med Mol Imaging. 2018;45(5):846–59.

39. Finlay IG, Mason MD, Shelley M. Radioisotopes for the palliation of metastatic bone cancer: a systematic review. Lancet Oncol. 2005;6:392–400.

40. Collins C, Eary JF, Donaldson G, Vernon C, Bush NE, Petersdorf S, et al. Samarium-153-EDTMP in bone metastases of hormone refractory prostate carcinoma: a phase I/II trial. J Nucl Med. 1993;34:1839–44.

41. Paszkowski AL, Hewitt DJ, Taylor AJR. Disseminated intravascular coagulation in a patient treated with strontium-89 for metastatic carcinoma of the prostate. Clin Nucl Med. 1999;24:852–4.

42. Wood TJ, Racano A, Yeung H, Farrokhyar F, Ghert M, Deheshi BM. Surgical management of bone metastases: quality of evidence and systematic review. Ann Surg Oncol. 2014;21(13):4081–9.

43. Roque M, Martinez MJ, Alonso P, Catala E, Garcia JL, Ferrandiz M. Radioisotopes for metastatic bone pain. Cochrane Database Syst Rev. 2003;4:CD003347.

44. Bauman G, Charette M, Reid R, Sathya J. Radiopharmaceuticals for the palliation of painful bone metastasis—a systemic review. Radiother Oncol. 2005;75:258–70.

45. D'Angelo G, Sciuto R, Salvatori M, Sperduti I, Mantini G, Maini CL, et al. Targeted "bone-seeking" radiopharmaceuticals for palliative treatment of bone metastases: a systematic review and meta-analysis. Q J Nucl Med Mol Imaging. 2012;56:538–43.

46. Serafini AN, Houston SJ, Resche I, Quick DP, Grund FM, Ell PJ, et al. Palliation of pain associated with metastatic bone cancer using samarium-153 lexidronam: a double-blind placebo-controlled clinical trial. J Clin Oncol. 1998;16(4):1574.

47. Sartor O, Reid RH, Hoskin PJ, Quick DP, Ell PJ, Coleman RE, et al. Samarium-153-Lexidronam complex for treatment of painful bone metastases in hormone-refractory prostate cancer. Urology. 2004;63(5):940.

48. Christensen MH, Petersen LJ. Radionuclide treatment of painful bone metastases in patients with breast cancer: a systematic review. Cancer Treat Rev. 2012;38:164–71.

49. Resche I, Chatal JF, Pecking A, Ell P, Duchesne G, Rubens R, et al. A dose-controlled study of 153Sm-ethylenediaminetetramethylenephosphonate (EDTMP) in the treatment of patients with painful bone metastases. Eur J Cancer. 1997;33:1583–91.

50. Baczyk M, Czepczynski R, Milecki P, Pisarek M, Oleksa R, Sowinski J. 89Sr versus 153Sm-EDTMP: comparison of treatment efficacy of painful bone metastases in prostate and breast carcinoma. Nucl Med Commun. 2007;28:245–50.

51. Kurosaka S, Satoh T, Chow E, Asano Y, Tabata K, Kimura M, et al. EORTC QLQ-BM22 and QLQ-C30 quality of life scores in patients with painful bone metastases of prostate cancer treated with strontium-89 radionuclide therapy. Ann Nucl Med. 2012;26:485–91.

52. Porter AT, McEwan AJ, Powe JE, Reid R, McGowan DG, Lukka H, et al. Results of a randomized phase-III trial to evaluate the efficacy of strontium-89 adjuvant to local field external beam irradiation in the management of endocrine resistant metastatic prostate cancer. Int J Radiat Oncol Biol Phys. 1993;25:805–13.

53. Tu SM, Millikan RE, Mengistu B, Delpassand ES, Amato RJ, Pagliaro LC, et al. Bone-targeted therapy for advanced androgen-independent carcinoma of the prostate: a randomised phase II trial. Lancet. 2001;357:336–41.

54. Smeland S, Erikstein B, Aas M, Skovlund E, Hess SL, Fossa SD. Role of strontium-89 as adjuvant to palliative external beam radiotherapy is questionable: results of a double-blind randomized study. Int J Radiat Oncol Biol Phys. 2003;56:1397–404.

55. James ND, Pirrie SJ, Pope AM, Barton D, Andronis L, Goranitis I, et al. Clinical outcomes and survival following treatment of metastatic castrate-refractory prostate cancer with docetaxel alone or with strontium-89, zoledronic acid, or both: the TRAPEZE randomized clinical trial. JAMA Oncol. 2016;2(4):493.

56. Lam MGEH, Dahmane A, Stevens WHM, van Rijk PP, de Klerk JMH, Zonnenberg BA. Combined use of zoledronic acid and 153Sm-EDTMP in hormone-refractory prostate cancer patients with bone metastases. Eur J Nucl Med Mol Imaging. 2008;35:756–65.

57. Storto G, Klain M, Paone G, Liuzzi R, Molino L, Marinelli A, et al. Combined therapy of Sr-89 and zoledronic acid in patients with painful bone metastases. Bone. 2006;39:35–41.

58. Rasulova N, Lyubshin V, Arybzhanov D, Sagdullaev S, Krylov V, Khodjibekov M. Optimal timing of bisphosphonate administration in combination with samarium-153 oxabifore in the treatment of painful metastatic bone disease. World J Nucl Med. 2013;12:14–8.

59. Henkin RE, Del Rowe JD, Grigsby PW, Hartford AC, Jadvar H, Macklis RM, et al. ACR-ASTRO practice guideline for the performance of therapy with unsealed radiopharmaceutical sources. Clin Nucl Med. 2011;36(8):e72–80.

60. Eary JF, Collins C, Stabin M, Vernon C, Petersdorf S, Baker M, et al. Samarium-153-EDTMP biodistribution and dosimetry estimation. J Nucl Med. 1993;34:1031–6.

61. Taylor AJ Jr. Strontium-89 for the palliation of bone pain due to metastatic disease. J Nucl Med. 1994;35:2054.

62. Silberstein EB, Williams C. Strontium-89 therapy for the pain of osseous metastases. J Nucl Med. 1985;26:345–8.

Selective Internal Radiotherapy (SIRT) of Primary Hepatic Carcinoma and Liver Metastases

7

Niklaus Schaefer

7.1 Introduction

SIRT (selective internal radiation therapy) is a form of internal radiation given to a selective site. In Nuclear Medicine the term "SIRT" is usually used in the context of internal radiation of liver metastases and primary liver tumors as HCC. Other terms for this form of treatment are liver radioembolization or trans-arterial radioembolization (TARE).

All forms of intra-arterial treatments of liver tumors have a distinctive mode of action. The liver is perfused by the liver arteries and the portal vein. In physiological condition the liver is perfused around 90% by the portal vein, and around 10% by the hepatic arteries. In contrast, intrahepatic tumors are normally perfused only by the arterial vessels and therefore restricted from the portal venous flow (Fig. 7.1). Therefore, catheterizing the arterial blood flow is of specific interest since different forms of payload can be transported in the tumoral capillary bed. Several forms of intra-arterial liver-directed treatments exist. The trans-arterial embolization (TAE) is used to obliterate the arterial supply of liver primary tumors or liver metastases. TAE or bland embolization of intrahepatic arteries aims to block the hepatic arterial flow using different embolic agents to induce ischemia. The trans-arterial chemotherapy (TACE) consists of a chemotherapeutic agent mixed with an embolic material. This combination allows a very high concentration of chemotherapy in the respective metastases. A third relatively widely used therapy option is the trans-arterial radioembolization. Contrary to TAE and TACE it deposits radiation in the tumor bed and can be used in patients who develop chemo-resistant metastases. Furthermore it is in contrary to TAE and TACE not embolic. TARE therefore has less complication, is overall better tolerated by the patients, and can be used in larger tumor burden in the liver. In the following chapter we overview technical aspects, the dosimetry, clinical data, side effects, and how to follow up patients after TARE.

7.2 Technical Procedure

A TARE procedure consists of two major technical sessions, which are performed, by a radiologist and nuclear physician in consensus. It needs to be underlined that the nuclear physician needs a profound understanding of the liver anatomy to understand angiography images and possible pitfalls, as well as the radiologist needs the knowledge about the nuclear medicine procedure and interpretation of the functional images. It is also mandated that the NM physician and the radiologist both perform a pre-interventional visit to discuss the indication and possible contraindications

N. Schaefer (✉)
Department of Nuclear Medicine, University Hospital of Lausanne, Lausanne, Switzerland
e-mail: Niklaus.Schaefer@chuv.ch

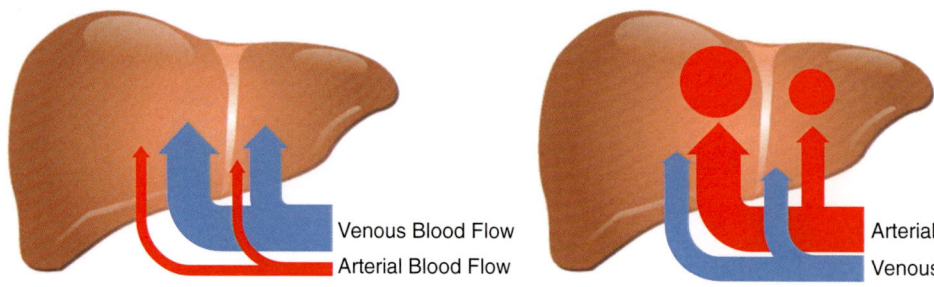

Fig. 7.1 General principle of hepatic blood flow in a normal liver and a liver with tumor metastases or primary tumors

Table 7.1 Contraindication for Liver TARE

• Ascites or other clinical signs of liver failure on physical exam [absolute]
• Pregnancy [absolute]
• Previous radiation therapy to the liver (not stereotactic, gamma/cyberknife)
• Excessive tumor burden with limited hepatic reserve (>66%)
• Capecitabine within previous or subsequent 2 months
• Abnormal organ or bone marrow function as determined by:
– Total bilirubin level > 2.0 mg/dL (>34 μmol/L) in absence of reversible cause
– Serum albumin <3.0 g/dL
– AST (SGOT)/ALT (SGPT) >5 × institutional ULN
– Creatinine >2.5 mg/dL
– Platelets <60,000/μL; leukocytes <2500/μL; absolute neutrophil <1500/μL
Following work-up procedure:
• Pre-treatment scan showing >20% Lung Shunting [absolute]
• Non-correctable shunting to the GI tract [absolute]

(Table 7.1) of the patient and discuss all cases in the multidisciplinary tumor board to evaluate all possible therapy option for the patient.

After decision to perform a TARE and obtained consensus of the patient two principal interventional session need to be planned (Fig. 7.2). A first session is purely diagnostic and establishes the principle knowledge about the anatomic properties of the arterial perfusion using the angiography. In this first session possible interfering arteries, for example, gastric or duodenal arteries, might need coiling by the radiologist to avoid misplacement of the radioactive beads in the therapy session. After careful analy-

sis of the arterial perfusion of the liver, an injection of Tc99m macro-albumins (MAA) is performed at the respective site where the therapeutic injection is anticipated. The dose of Tc99m MAA might be prescribed between 60 MBq for a single left lobe and 180 MBq for an injection of the total liver.

After successful injection of Tc99m MAA, the patient should be transferred with not too much delay in the Nuclear Medicine unit to perform scintigraphy to avoid free technetium-99m in the diagnostic images. Usually the diagnostic scintigraphy scan aims to calculate the liver-versus-lung ratio to calculate a possible shunting of the MAA product in liver veins and subsequently in the lung. A shunt up to 10% needs no therapy adaption, if shunt is between 10% and 20% a dose reduction is anticipated and a shunt >20% needs either replanning of the angiography to exclude the shunting liver volume or the patient cannot be treated by TARE. After planar liver / thorax imaging, usually a single photon computed tomography (SPECT) of the liver region needs to be performed. The SPECT identifies visually and computationally the ratio between malignant liver tumors and normal liver tissue which needs to be spared from internal radiation. As general rule the radiation applied to the normal liver should not exceed 40 Gy to avoid liver fibrosis. However this limit has been set using external beam radiation and is the limit to induce liver fibrosis of the normal liver. Newer data recommend doses for the normal liver up to 70 Gy. Further careful evaluation needs to be performed on intestinal shunting, for example, in the duodenal/pyloric region, the gastric wall, and the pancreas. After evaluating the above parameter, a

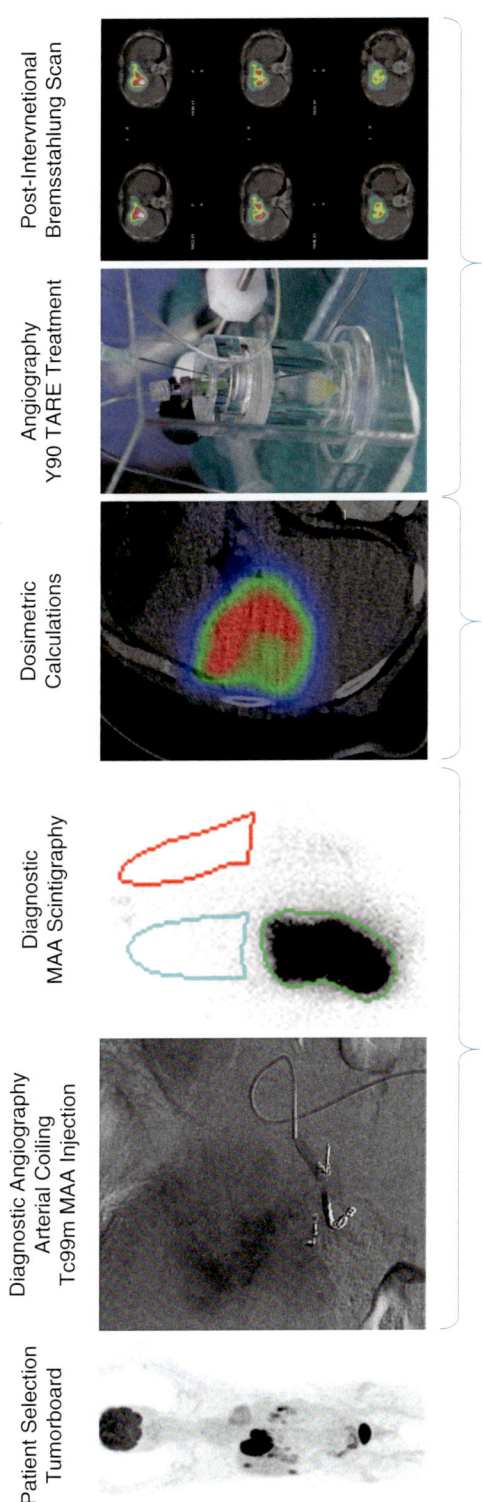

Fig. 7.2 Workflow of a TARE procedure

dosimetry to optimize the given dose is recommended and the patient is planned for the therapeutic procedure. This second intervention usually is planned at a different day after performing dose calculation or dosimetry. The principle of dose calculation and dosimetry is described in the next section.

The therapeutic procedure needs again careful investigation of the liver arterial anatomy. Due to coiling of relevant arteries the arterial perfusion, for example, of the duodenum, via a supra-duodenal artery or any other intestinal organs might change. After careful investigation the catheter is placed at the respective site of the preparation scan and the infusion of the radioactive, therapeutic beads is performed by the radiologist and nuclear physician in consensus. There are two general therapeutic products used for the TARE procedure (Table 7.2) which both are based on the Y90 isotope. Y90 is a relatively strong radiating isotope (T1/2 64.10 h; β⁻ energy 2282 MeV). It is therefore very important that the staff is securely protected at all tasks and the procedure is supervised by personnel trained in radiation safety. Furthermore the angiography room needs to be approved for open unsealed radioactive sources.

After infusions of the Y90 beads, the patient is transferred to the nuclear medicine unit to perform a bremsstrahlung scan using SPECT imaging or an Y90 PET/CT to confirm the distribution of the internal radiation (Fig. 7.3). The patient furthermore needs carful clinical investigation to exclude short-term significant side effects (Table 7.2). A control by the referring physician is recommended in the first two weeks to exclude further side effects. Imaging control is recommended usually after three months and will be discussed later in the text.

7.3 Dose Calculation and Dosimetry

The dose calculation relies on the simple principle not to harm the normal liver tissue caused by off target treatment and lung tissue caused by arteriovenous shunting of the radioactive spheres. It has been shown in the past that patients receiving more than 40 Gy on the normal liver by external beam radiation develop radiation-induced liver fibrosis (REILD). REILD is a subacute form of liver injury and develops usually after 4 weeks or later. The symptoms of a REILD are usually fatigue and right upper quadrant pain. Physician examination can resemble a Budd-Chiari syndrome with ascites and jaundice. A radiation-induced lung disease might develop in patients receiving over 20 Gy external beam radiation. There are several methods to calculate a dose for patients receiving a selective internal radiotherapy. Most simple is a body surface method, which takes the affected liver versus normal liver into account. This method is called the BSA model (body surface area). It is a validated method to prescribe a dose; however, due to a calculation using a ratio this model is sensitive for overtreatment in small livers with small tumors and under treatment in large livers with large tumors.

7.3.1 BSA Formula

$$DOSE(GBq) = BSA(m2)$$
$$- 0.2 + \left(\frac{Volume_{Tumor}}{Volume_{Tumor} + Volume_{Liver}} \right)$$

The BSA formula has been mainly developed for SIR Spheres treatment and is still currently used by many centers. The calculation for the Therasphere product is different. The recommended dose by the producer is between 80 Gy and 150 Gy. The amount of radioactivity required to deliver the desired dose to the liver may be calculated using the following formula:

Table 7.2 Products used for Liver TARE

	Glass (TheraSphere)	Resin (SIR Spheres)
Size	20–30 μm	20–60 μm
Isotope	Yttrium-90 in glass matrix	Yttrium-90 on resin surface
Specific gravity	High	Low
Activity/sphere (at calibration)	2500 Bq	50 Bq
# of dose sizes	6 (3, 5, 7, 10, 15, 20 GBq)	1 (3 GBq)
# spheres/dose	1.2–8 Million	40–80 Million
# spheres/3GBq dose	1.2 Million	40–80 Million

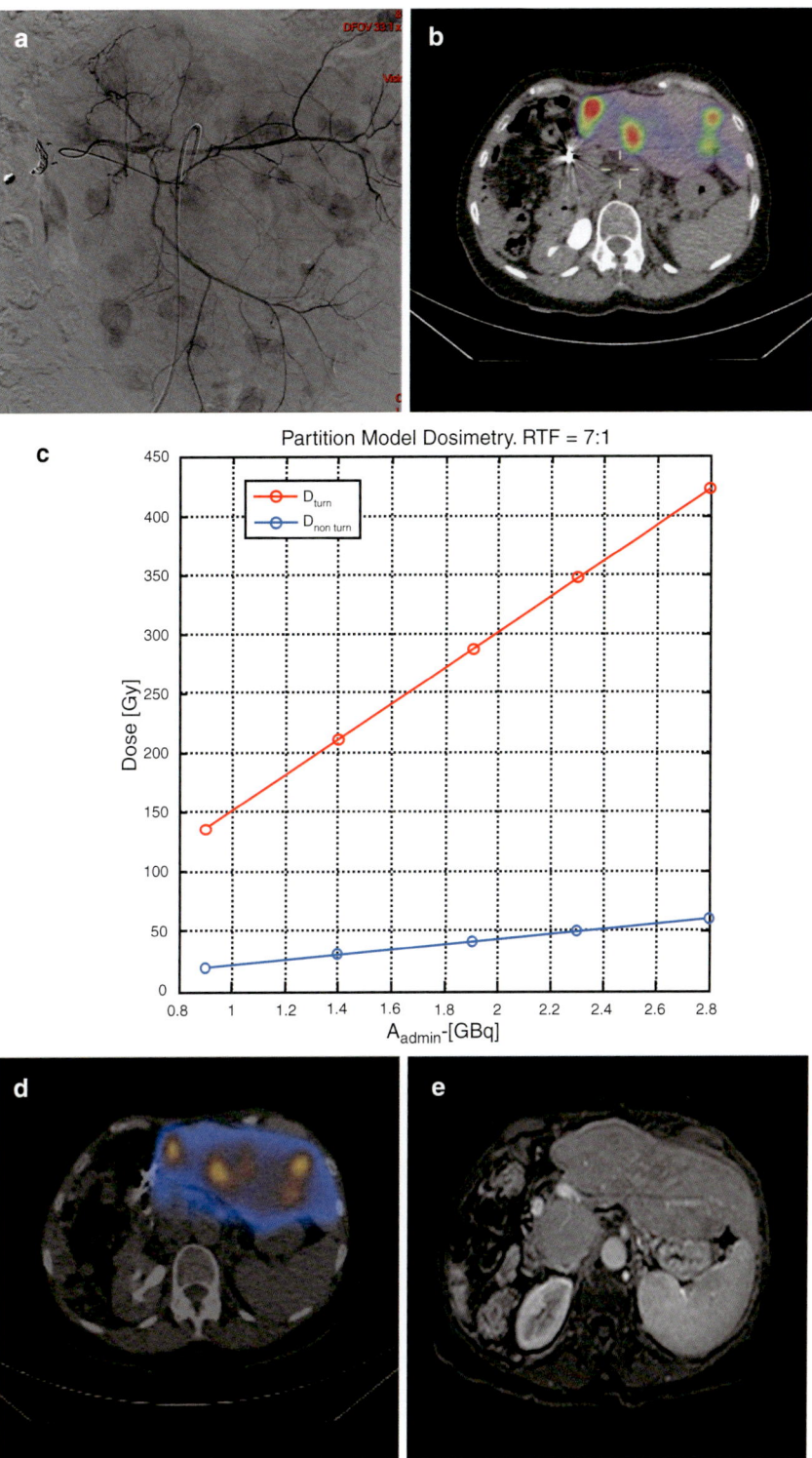

Fig. 7.3 (**a**) Angiography of a patient with well-differentiated NET, post right hemi-hepatectomy showing multiple liver lesions in the remaining left lobe. (**b**) SPECT/CT after injection of 60 MBq of ^{99m}Tc loaded macroalbumines. (**c**) Partition model dose estimation: (blue) normal liver, (red) tumoral liver. Predicting a dose of 40 Gy to the normal left liver and 270 Gy on the metastatic NET lesions using a dose of 1.8 GBq of Y90 TARE. (**d**) SPECT/CT after 1.8 GBq of Y90 TARE. (**e**) Follow-up MRI showing a very favorable response

$$Activity\,(GBq) = \left(Desired\,Dose_{Gy}\right) * \frac{Mass\,of\,Targeted\,Liver_{kg}}{50*\left(1-Lung\,Shunt\,Fraction\right)}$$

It is highly recommended that TARE dosing is performed by a highly experienced Nuclear Medicine specialist or a dedicated physicist. The compartment partition model is the most accurate means to determine the dose administered to the liver tumor, the normal parenchyma, and the lung and is based on uptake ratios, liver tumor volumetry, normal liver volumetry, and lung uptake [1].

7.4   Clinical Data

7.4.1   Hepatocellular Carcinoma (HCC)

HCC is a primary carcinoma of the liver and therefore is very suitable for liver-directed treatments. However, especially in limited disease many options exist and the indication to either operate, radiofrequency, TACE (trans-arterial chemoembolization) or SIRT versus systemic treatment options have to be discussed carefully in a dedicated tumor board together with hepatologists, surgeons, interventional radiologists, oncologists and nuclear physicians. Guidance can be given via different staging systems, however in HCC the Barcelona criteria (BCLC) are of use for treatment guidance. TARE has been tested in early BCLC A to advanced stages (BCLC C). Importantly, TARE has been shown to be safe in patients with portal venous thrombosis (PVT).

The efficacy of TARE in HCC is highly dependent on a number of factors regarding liver function, patient performance status, and tumor extension (BCLC, UNOS, Child-Pugh). First series published by the Northwestern group reported in 291 patients and 526 TARE treatments and overall time to progression of 7.9 months and an overall survival differed between patients with Child-Pugh A and B disease (A, 17.2 months; B, 7.7 months; $p = 0.002$). Patients with Child-Pugh B disease who had portal vein thrombosis (PVT) survived 5.6 months (95% confidence interval,

4.5–6.7) [2]. A multicenter study by Sangro et al. reported outcome of TARE in 325 HCC patients. The consortium reported a median overall survival of 12.8 months in the overall population. Divided in subgroups according to BCLC stages, outcome by disease stage (BCLC A 24.4 months; BCLC B 16.9 month; BCLC C 10.0 months) [95% CI, 7.7–10.9 months]. Reported prognostic factors in this study were ECOG status, hepatic function (Child-Pugh class, ascites, and baseline total bilirubin), tumor burden (number of nodules, alpha-fetoprotein), and presence of extrahepatic disease [3]. Very recent prospective and randomized studies compare the efficacy of TARE versus systemic treatment. A large European study showed no difference in overall survival of TARE versus Sorafenib (Beyer Pharma, Berlin Germany). In brief, overall 467 patients were investigated and randomized into the TARE or Sorafenib group. Median overall survival was 8.0 months in the TARE group versus 9.9 months in the Sorafenib group ($p = 0.18$) [4]. However, patients undergoing a single TARE intervention had significant less toxicities than patients in the Sorafenib group. This trial was paired by a HCC trial in the Asia-Pacific region. Patients coming from this region have a distinct different survival due to much more underlying viral hepatitis as disease driver. Overall, this trial compared the safety and efficacy of Asian patients receiving either Sorafenib or TARE. Median OS was 8.8–10.0 months with TARE and Sorafenib, respectively (hazard ratio, 1.1; 95% CI, 0.9–1.4; $p = 0.36$) and therefore revealed no significant difference. However, TARE was significantly better tolerated [5]. There are several ongoing trials to prospectively investigate the role of SIRT in advanced HCC patients. A very prominent study is the STOP HCC trial by the Northwestern group, which might be the largest multicenter study looking again at the question of Sorafenib and TARE as first line in HCC patients [6].

Another important questions is to bridge patients to liver transplantation has been recently investigated. This might be a very useful concept since patients usually wait long term to receive a donor liver. A recent combined series of 178 patients revealed promising data for patients with HCC waiting for liver transplant [7]. Further concept involves liver TARE prior to hemihepatectomy to induce liver growth in the future liver remnant (FLR). It has been shown that FLR growth after TARE reaches around 50% after nine months [8]. Other studies investigate the efficacy of TARE against TACE in HCC. Among somewhat heterogeneous study results, large centers have shown that partial response rates favor TARE-Y90 versus TACE (61% vs. 37%) and downstaging to UNOS T2 was achieved in 58% of the TARE patients compared to 31% of TACE patients [9]. Further studies investigated the role of surgery in HCC post-TARE. Very recent studies show the safety and efficacy of combining TARE and surgery [10].

Overall TARE in HCC seems to be a very useful therapy option. However, prospective studies in a rather unselected patient population have not shown superiority of TARE versus Sorafenib. This underlines the importance how to choose correctly the patients and the necessity that all patients need to be performed at large center and have to be evaluated by a dedicated tumor board.

7.4.2 Metastatic Colon Cancer (mCRC)

The liver is a predominant site of distant metastases in patients with advanced colon cancer. In the last twenty years, the evolution of systemic chemotherapy combined with antibody treatment in selected patients did yield high response rates and prolonged overall survival. In this rapidly evolving therapeutic armamentarium TARE treatment needs to be chosen with care. In general, the same rule as for HCC applies. All patients need to be seen in a dedicated colorectal tumor board with all respective specialists. Especially the oncologists need to exclude useful systemic therapies prior to set an indication for TARE in mCRC,

since we speak, in contrast to HCC, of metastasized disease once liver tumor occur.

Early randomized data compared TARE in combination with floxuridine versus floxuridine only. Progression-free survival was significantly linger in patients receiving TARE (15.9 vs. 9.7 months, p = 0.001) and toxicity was reported to be very low without grade 3 or 4 toxicity. A phase III study by Flamen et al. tested TARE in combination with 5 fluorouracil (5-FU) vs. 5-FU only. Median time to progression was significantly longer in the TARE group (2.1 vs. 5.5 months; p = 0.003) and median overall survival was 7.3 vs. 10.0 months in the TARE group [11]. A phase I study by Sharma et al. evaluated the combination of TARE with a modern FOLFOX (5-FU, Oxaliplatin) regime. In this study 20 patients were enrolled and 18 of 20 patients showed a partial response in the further evaluation. Median progression-free survival was 9.3 months, and median time to progression in the liver was 12.3 months. The dose-limiting toxicity was neutropenia but the combination was in general well tolerated [12]. The promising results of this phase I study led to the design of a large phase III study to test TARE combined with FOLFOX versus FOLFOX alone. In a large patient population the median PFS at any site was 10.2 vs. 10.7 months in TARE plus FOLFOX versus FOLFOX alone (p = 0.43). However, the liver only PFS revealed a significant longer local PFS of 20.5 vs. 12.6 months (p = 0.002). Higher grade adverse events were reported in 73.4–85.4% of patients in FOLFOX versus the combined group [13]. This data has been pooled with the FOXFIRE trial [14] and global results were reported in over 1000 patients. Although higher numbers in patients, the addition of SIRT to first-line FOLFOX chemotherapy for patients with liver-only and liver-dominant metastatic colorectal cancer did not improve overall survival compared with that for FOLFOX alone [15]. Altogether, SIRT in combination with FOLFOX cannot be recommended in early treatment lines. A current study (EPOCH, TS-102 study) is currently evaluating TARE in combination with standard of care chemotherapy in second line [16]. Overlooking the current evidence how to implement TARE in the treatment of mCRC it is recommended to evaluate all validated systemic therapy in a tumor board setting prior to treat with TARE. Currently TARE is well accepted as salvage treatment in patients with liver-dominant disease.

7.4.3 Metastatic Neuroendocrine Tumors (mNET)

NET are a variety of tumors with endocrine features originating from the neural crest. In general, NET are divided in foregut, midgut, hindgut, and pancreatic neuroendocrine tumors. Although well differentiated in many cases, NET tend to metastasize in lymph nodes, bone, and liver and are due to their slow progression identified usually at a later stage. In the case of metastasized NET, many options exist and are dependent on the primary site and the mitotic level (Ki-67) of the tumor. Therefore all NET patients need to be discussed in a dedicated neuroendocrine tumor board with NET specialists and only in very specific cases TARE might be an option.

Many phase II studies have already been published. The largest series by Kennedy showed stable disease in 22.7%, partial response in 60.5%, complete in 2.7%, and progressive disease in 4.9% of the NET patients. In the treated patient population no radiation liver failure occurred and the median survival was reported to be 70 months [17]. A more recent study by Peker et al. demonstrated the safety and effectiveness for the treatment of unresectable liver NETs with one- and two-year survival rates of 71% and 45%, respectively [18]. A meta-analysis revealed an objective response of 50% and a weighted average DCR of 86%. This large meta-analysis considered TARE as effective treatment option for patients with hepatic metastatic NET with high response rates and survival.

7.4.4 Metastatic Breast Cancer (mBCa)

Metastatic breast cancer patients have many systemic therapy options. Prior to any locoregional therapy they have to be carefully evaluated at the dedicated tumor board to exclude useful systemic options. Furthermore, these patients were sometimes under chemotherapy and anti-hormonal therapy for many years. Therefore the liver reserve might be limited and the patients have to be treated with special care and possible dose reduction.

There is no prospective TARE data in mBCa patients. An early study by Salem et al. investigated 27 patients with complete and partial response in 39.1% patients (in nine patients), stable disease in 52.1% patients, and progressive disease in 8.8% patients. Despite this response rates, the median survival was only several months [19]. This trial shows exemplary that mBCa has to be seen as systemic disease and the role of locoregional treatments needs to be further explored. In the recent years larger retrospective studies have been published. A study by Fendler et al. reported a response rate of 52% in FDG—PET after TARE, leading to a median overall survival of 35 weeks [20].

7.4.5 Melanoma

Melanoma has to be divided into ocular melanoma (OM) which has a strong liver tropism and therefore is a suitable target for TARE versus a melanoma originating from the skin leading to metastases at many different sites. Currently many new therapy options, especially in the field of immunotherapy, evolve. Therefore these patients have to be discussed in the respective tumor board prior to any locoregional procedure.

A recent study of TARE in OM showed a hepatic progression-free survival of 5.9 months and an overall survival of 12.3 months. The median overall survival after diagnosis of liver metastases was 23.9 months [21]. In this salvage patient population these numbers seem encouraging. A very recent report of a nationwide analysis of TARE in OM showed tumor control in overall 61% of the patients. The median overall survival was 18.7 months [22].

7.4.6 Intrahepatic Cholangiocarcinoma (iCC)

ICC is a primary liver tumor evolving from the small bile ducts. In contrast to HCC these tumors are usually less arterialized and therefore less suitable for intra-arterial therapies. Nevertheless, several studies have been published to investigate TARE in this patient population.

Earlier studies by Lewandowski et al. showed partial response in 25%, stable disease in 73%, and progressive disease in 2% of the patients [23]. A very recent study reported a median overall survival of 21.4 months after initial diagnosis and 12.0 months after TARE. Especially patients with solitary tumors have good outcome with an overall survival of 25 months after performing TARE [24]. Overlooking current data, TARE might be an interesting therapy option for patients with iCC, who have normally limited therapy options.

7.5   Follow-Up Imaging

Follow-up imaging after liver-directed radioembolization (TARE) is always a challenge. Main problems are the inflammatory changes after high-dose radiation and generally delayed anatomic response to TARE. Early literature compared anatomical imaging by computed tomography (CT) against metabolic imaging by FDG—PET. A reduction in metabolic activity measured by SUVmax precedes the anatomical size reduction [25] in metastatic colorectal cancer (mCRC). Other series in mixed histologies confirmed this finding where FDG—PET detected responders 6 weeks after intervention [26] where only 13% of these patients did show reduction in size (PR) in the anatomical imaging. More recent studies confirmed the prognostic role of early FDG—PET in mCRC after TARE. Four weeks after the intervention, a reduction of SUVmax of at least 50% predicted a difference in survival of 10 months versus 4 months in mCRC [27]. Identical results were published in HCC, where metabolic responders survived 10 months versus non-responders who did survive only 5 months [28]. Further studies supported the evidence in metastatic breast cancer, where post-treatment FDG—PET three months after TARE was the only independent predictor of the survival outcome (65 weeks vs 43 weeks; $p < 0.05$) [29]. In patients with intrahepatic cholangiocarcinoma, a reduction of FDG avidity predicted outcome where responders had a survival of 114 weeks versus 19 weeks in non-responders [30]. More recently,

advanced response criteria (PERCIST) have been evaluated to assess response in TARE patients. Change in SUVpeak and total lesions glycolysis predicted overall survival ($p = 0.039$; hazard ratio [HR], 0.24; 95% confidence interval [CI], 0.06–0.93), progression-free survival ($p = 0.016$; HR, 0.15; 95% CI, 0.03–0.69), and time to intrahepatic progression ($p = 0.010$; HR, 0.16; 95% CI, 0.04–0.65). Interestingly, in the same study summed baseline CT diameter of less than 8 cm for the 2 largest liver metastases predicted time to intrahepatic progression ($p = 0.013$; HR, 0.21; 95% CI, 0.06–0.72) but did not predict overall or progression-free survival [31]. Overall, the body of evidence supports that a reduction of FDG avidity in early PET (4 weeks) might be useful to predict further outcome of the patients. Not many early studies investigated the role of MRI in the follow-up after TARE. Enhancement around a treated lesion after TARE is a finding often observed in MRI, corresponding to the inflammation area of the hepatic parenchyma and sometimes misunderstood as tumor viability or tumor progression. A recent comparison of FDG—PET and DWI—MRI before and 6 weeks after TARE showed a higher positive predictive and a higher negative predictive value for DWI—MRI versus FDG—PET (96% vs. 88%; 96% vs. 56%). Overall, the detection for response was higher for DWI—MRI than for FDG—PET/CT (96%; 22/23 vs. 65%; 15/23) ($p < 0.02$) [32]. Overall, more recent studies show the value of DWI—MRI and the paradigm that early FDG—PET best detects outcome might be questioned. As pointed out, early studies showed the superiority of functional PET imaging to CT. One major problem is certainly, that in general, RECIST criteria are not suitable for modern treatments. This problem was already identified in patients undergoing anti-angiogenesis treatment, as, for example, SORAFENIB in HCC [33]. A recent study investigating different criteria found that RECIST 1.1 after TARE is not suitable to assess response in these patients. However, the same study found Choi criteria and difference in tumor attenuation well predicts outcome in TARE mCRC patients and has the same predictive power as the EORTC PET response criteria [34]. Overall, the paradigm that CT might not be an imaging of choice has to be re-challenged in the light of new response criteria and more advanced protocols as arterial perfusion protocols. An interesting approach is to predict survival outcome by measuring relative or absolute radiation dose targeted to the tumor lesions by Bremsstrahlung SPECT/CT or PET/CT. Lam et al. showed that the Y90 Bremsstrahlung PET might predict further outcome in non-resectable mCRC patients undergoing the TARE procedure [35].

7.6 Outlook in the Future

Currently TARE is performed using Y90 bound resin or glass micropsheres. Future compounds might use other isotopes as Holmium-166 (Quirem Microspheres, Quirem Medical BV, The Netherlands). The advantage of this procedure is the visibility of Holmuim-166 in the MRI scan [36]. This might facilitate therapy planning. However, further prospective trials have to investigate the role of Holmium-166 Spheres versus Glass and Resin Y90 based microspheres.

7.7 Conclusion

TARE is a highly effective and safe procedure; however, it has to be used in the right patient at the right time. Most recent data have disappointed the community since it has been shown that Y90 microsphere treatment cannot be used in an unselected patient population, for example, in HCC or mCRC. It is therefore highly important that we further investigate the role of TARE in different indication to explore the right use of this promising technique.

References

1. Gulec SA, Mesoloras G, Stabin M. Dosimetric techniques in 90Y-microsphere therapy of liver cancer: the MIRD equations for dose calculations. J Nucl Med. 2006;47:1209–11.
2. Salem R, Lewandowski RJ, Mulcahy MF, Riaz A, Ryu RK, Ibrahim S, Kulik L, et al. Radioembolization for hepatocellular carcinoma using yttrium-90 microspheres: a comprehensive report of long-term outcomes. Gastroenterology. 2010;138(1):52–64. https://doi.org/10.1053/j.gastro.2009.09.006.
3. Sangro B, Carpanese L, Cianni R, Golfieri R, Gasparini D, Ezziddin S, et al. Survival after yttrium-90 resin microsphere radioembolization of hepatocellular carcinoma across Barcelona clinic liver cancer stages: a European evaluation. Hepatology. 2011;54(3):868–78. https://doi.org/10.1002/hep.24451.
4. Vilgrain V, Pereira H, Assenat E, Guiu B, Ilonca AD, Pageaux G-P, Marthey L, et al. Efficacy and safety of selective internal radiotherapy with yttrium-90 resin microspheres compared with sorafenib in locally advanced and inoperable hepatocellular carcinoma (SARAH): an open-label randomised controlled phase 3 trial. Lancet Oncol. 2017;18(12):1624–36. https://doi.org/10.1016/s1470-2045(17)30683-6.
5. Chow PKH, Gandhi M, Tan S-B, Khin MW, Khasbazar A, Ong J, et al. SIRveNIB: Selective internal radiation therapy versus sorafenib in Asia-pacific patients with hepatocellular carcinoma. J Clin Oncol. 2018;36(19):1913–21. https://doi.org/10.1200/jco.2017.76.0892.
6. Chauhan N, Bukovcan J, Boucher E, Cosgrove D, Edeline J, Hamilton B, Salem R, et al. Intra-arterial therasphere yttrium-90 glass microspheres in the treatment of patients with unresectable hepatocellular carcinoma: protocol for the STOP-HCC phase 3 randomized controlled trial. JMIR Res Protoc. 2018;7(8):e11234. https://doi.org/10.2196/11234.
7. Levi Sandri GB, Ettorre GM, Giannelli V, Colasanti M, Sciuto R, Pizzi G, Lucatelli P, et al. Trans-arterial radio-embolization: a new chance for patients with hepatocellular cancer to access liver transplantation, a world review. Transl Gastroenterol Hepatol. 2017;2(11):98. https://doi.org/10.21037/tgh.2017.11.11.
8. Vouche M, Lewandowski RJ, Atassi R, Memon K, Gates VL, Ryu RK, Salem R, et al. Radiation lobectomy: time-dependent analysis of future liver remnant volume in unresectable liver cancer as a bridge to resection. J Hepatol. 2013;59(5):1029–36. https://doi.org/10.1016/j.jhep.2013.06.015.
9. Lewandowski RJ, Kulik LM, Riaz A, Senthilnathan S, Mulcahy MF, Ryu RK, Salem R, et al. A comparative analysis of transarterial downstaging for hepatocellular carcinoma: chemoembolization versus radioembolization. Am J Transplant. 2009;9(8):1920–8. https://doi.org/10.1111/j.1600-6143.2009.02695.x.
10. Gabr A, Abouchaleh N, Ali R, Baker T, Caicedo J, Katariya N, Salem R, et al. Outcomes of surgical resection after radioembolization for hepatocellular carcinoma. J Vasc Interv Radiol. 2018;29(11):1502–1510.e1. https://doi.org/10.1016/j.jvir.2018.06.027.
11. Hendlisz A, Van den Eynde M, Peeters M, Maleux G, Lambert B, Vannoote J, Flamen P, et al. Phase III trial comparing protracted intravenous fluorouracil infusion alone or with yttrium-90 resin microspheres radioembolization for liver-limited metastatic colorectal cancer refractory to standard chemotherapy. J Clin Oncol. 2010;28(23):3687–94. https://doi.org/10.1200/jco.2010.28.5643.
12. Sharma RA, Van Hazel GA, Morgan B, Berry DP, Blanshard K, Price D, Steward WP, et al.

Radioembolization of liver metastases from colorectal cancer using yttrium-90 microspheres with concomitant systemic oxaliplatin, fluorouracil, and leucovorin chemotherapy. J Clin Oncol. 2007;25(9):1099–106. https://doi.org/10.1200/jco.2006.08.7916.

13. van Hazel GA, Heinemann V, Sharma NK, Findlay MPN, Ricke J, Peeters M, Gibbs P, et al. SIRFLOX: randomized phase III trial comparing first-line mFOLFOX6 (Plus or Minus Bevacizumab) Versus mFOLFOX6 (Plus or Minus Bevacizumab) plus selective internal radiation therapy in patients with metastatic colorectal cancer. J Clin Oncol. 2016;34(15):1723–31. https://doi.org/10.1200/jco.2015.66.1181.

14. Dutton SJ, Kenealy N, Love SB, Wasan HS, Sharma RA. FOXFIRE protocol: an open-label, randomised, phase III trial of 5-fluorouracil, oxaliplatin and folinic acid (OxMdG) with or without interventional Selective Internal Radiation Therapy (SIRT) as first-line treatment for patients with unresectable liver-only or liver-dominant metastatic colorectal cancer. BMC Cancer. 2014;14(1):497. https://doi.org/10.1186/1471-2407-14-497.

15. Wasan HS, Gibbs P, Sharma NK, Taieb J, Heinemann V, Ricke J, Westcott M, et al. First-line selective internal radiotherapy plus chemotherapy versus chemotherapy alone in patients with liver metastases from colorectal cancer (FOXFIRE, SIRFLOX, and FOXFIRE-Global): a combined analysis of three multicentre, randomised, phase 3 trials. Lancet Oncol. 2017;18(9):1159–71. https://doi.org/10.1016/s1470-2045(17)30457-6.

16. Clinicaltrial.gov trial number : NCT01483027.

17. Kennedy AS, Dezarn WA, McNeillie P, Coldwell D, Nutting C, Carter D, Salem R, et al. Radioembolization for unresectable neuroendocrine hepatic metastases using resin 90Y-microspheres: early results in 148 patients. Am J Clin Oncol. 2008;31(3):271–9. https://doi.org/10.1097/coc.0b013e31815e4557.

18. Peker A, Çiçek O, Soydal Ç, Küçük NÖ, Bilgiç S. Radioembolization with yttrium-90 resin microspheres for neuroendocrine tumor liver metastases. Diagn Interv Radiol. 2015;21(1):54–9.

19. Bangash AK, Atassi B, Kaklamani V, Rhee TK, Yu M, Lewandowski RJ, Sato KT, Ryu RK, Gates VL, Newman S, Mandal R, Gradishar W, Omary RA, Salem R. 90Y radioembolization of metastatic breast cancer to the liver: toxicity, imaging response, survival. J Vasc Interv Radiol. 2007;18(5):621–8.

20. Fendler WP, Lechner H, Todica A, Paprotka KJ, Paprotka PM, Jakobs TF, Haug AR, et al. Safety, efficacy, and prognostic factors after radioembolization of hepatic metastases from breast cancer: a large single-center experience in 81 patients. J Nucl Med. 2016;57(4):517–23. https://doi.org/10.2967/jnumed.115.165050.

21. Eldredge-Hindy H, Ohri N, Anne PR, Eschelman D, Gonsalves C, Intenzo C, Sato T, et al. Yttrium-90 microsphere brachytherapy for liver metastases from uveal melanoma. Am J Clin Oncol. 2016;39(2):189–95. https://doi.org/10.1097/coc.0000000000000033.

22. Tulokas S, Mäenpää H, Peltola E, Kivelä T, Vihinen P, Virta A, Hernberg M, et al. Selective internal radiation therapy (SIRT) as treatment for hepatic metastases of uveal melanoma: a Finnish nation-wide retrospective experience. Acta Oncol. 2018;57(10):1373–80. https://doi.org/10.1080/0284186x.2018.1465587.

23. Mouli S, Memon K, Baker T, Benson AB III, Mulcahy MF, Gupta R, Lewandowski RJ, et al. Yttrium-90 radioembolization for intrahepatic cholangiocarcinoma: safety, response, and survival analysis. J Vasc Interv Radiol. 2013;24(8):1227–34. https://doi.org/10.1016/j.jvir.2013.02.031.

24. Gangi A, Shah J, Hatfield N, Smith J, Sweeney J, Choi J, Kis B, et al. Intrahepatic cholangiocarcinoma treated with transarterial yttrium-90 glass microsphere radioembolization: results of a single institution retrospective study. J Vasc Interv Radiol. 2018;29(8):1101–8. https://doi.org/10.1016/j.jvir.2018.04.001.

25. Lewandowski RJ, Thurston KG, Goin JE, et al. 90Y microsphere (TheraSphere) treatment for unresectable colorectal cancer metastases of the liver: response to treatment at targeted doses of 135-150 Gy as measured by [18F]fluorodeoxyglucose positron emission tomography and computed tomographic imaging. J Vasc Interv Radiol. 2005;16(12):1641–51.

26. Szyszko T, Al-Nahhas A, Canelo R, et al. Assessment of response to treatment of unresectable liver tumours with 90Y microspheres: value of FDG PET versus computed tomography. Nucl Med Commun. 2007;28(1):15–20.

27. Sabet A, Meyer C, Aouf A, et al. Early post-treatment FDG PET predicts survival after 90Y microsphere radioembolization in liver-dominant metastatic colorectal cancer. Eur J Nucl Med Mol Imaging. 2015;42(3):370–6.

28. Sabet A, Ahmadzadehfar H, Bruhman J, et al. Survival in patients with hepatocellular carcinoma treated with 90Y-microsphere radioembolization. Prediction by 18F-FDG PET. Nuklearmedizin. 2014;53(2):39–45. https://doi.org/10.3413/Nukmed-0622-13-09.

29. Haug AR, Tiega Donfack BP, Trumm C, et al. 18F-FDG PET/CT predicts survival after radioembolization of hepatic metastases from breast cancer. J Nucl Med. 2012;53(3):371–7.

30. Haug AR, Heinemann V, Bruns CJ, et al. 18F-FDG PET independently predicts survival in patients with cholangiocellular carcinoma treated with 90Y microspheres. Eur J Nucl Med Mol Imaging. 2011;38:1037–45.

31. Michl M, Lehner S, Paprottka PM, et al. Use of PERCIST for prediction of progression-free and overall survival after radioembolization for liver metastases from pancreatic cancer. J Nucl Med. 2016;57(3):355–60.

32. Barabasch A, Kraemer NA, Ciritsis A, et al. Diagnostic accuracy of diffusion-weighted magnetic resonance imaging versus positron emission tomography/computed tomography for early response assessment of liver metastases to Y90-radioembolization. Investig Radiol. 2015;50(6):409–15.

33. Edeline J, Boucher E, Rolland Y, et al. Comparison of tumor response by Response Evaluation Criteria in Solid Tumors (RECIST) and modified RECIST in patients treated with sorafenib for hepatocellular carcinoma. Cancer. 2012;118(1):147–56.

34. Shady W, Sotirchos VS, Do RK, et al. Surrogate imaging biomarkers of response of colorectal liver metastases after salvage radioembolization using 90Y-loaded resin microspheres. AJR Am J Roentgenol. 2016;207(3):661–70.

35. van den Hoven AF, Rosenbaum CE, Elias SG, et al. Insights into the dose-response relationship of radio-embolization with resin 90Y-microspheres: a prospective cohort study in patients with colorectal cancer liver metastases. J Nucl Med. 2016;57(7):1014–9.

36. Arranja AG, Hennink WE, Denkova AG, Hendrikx RWA, Nijsen JFW. Radioactive holmium phosphate microspheres for cancer treatment. Int J Pharm. 2018;548(1):73–81. https://doi.org/10.1016/j.ijpharm.2018.06.036.

Radioimmunotherapy of Lymphomas

8

Clément Bailly, Caroline Bodet-Milin, François Guerard, Nicolas Chouin, Joelle Gaschet, Michel Cherel, François Davodeau, Alain Faivre-Chauvet, Françoise Kraeber-Bodéré, and Mickaël Bourgeois

8.1 Introduction

Malignant lymphoma is a generic name describing a wide group of hematological cancers derived from white blood cells or lymphocytes. This group of pathologies presents a great variety of distinct diseases with heterogeneous histologic aspects, immunophenotypes, genetic abnormalities, and finally clinical outcomes for patients. The current 2016 WHO classification of mature lymphoid, histiocytic, and dendritic neoplasms differentiate lymphomas into mature B-cell neoplasms, mature T and NK neoplasms, Hodgkin lymphoma, posttransplant lymphoproliferative disorder (PTLD), and histiocytic and dendritic cell neoplasms [1]. Each of these lymphoma subtypes can be divided into histological subtypes as well as be separated according to their aggressive or indolent nature. In terms of frequencies, B-cell lymphoma is the most common at approximately

C. Bailly · C. Bodet-Milin · A. Faivre-Chauvet
F. Kraeber-Bodéré (✉)
INSERM UMR1232—CNRS UMR6299—Centre de Recherche en Cancérologie de Nantes-Angers (Equipe 13), Institut de Recherche en Santé de l'Université de Nantes, Nantes, France

Department of Nuclear Medicine, University Hospital, CHU de Nantes, Nantes, France
e-mail: clement.bailly@chu-nantes.fr;
caroline.milin@chu-nantes.fr;
alain.faivre-chauvet@univ-nantes.fr;
francoise.bodere@chu-nantes.fr

F. Guerard · J. Gaschet · F. Davodeau
INSERM UMR1232—CNRS UMR6299—Centre de Recherche en Cancérologie de Nantes-Angers (Equipe 13), Institut de Recherche en Santé de l'Université de Nantes, Nantes, France
e-mail: francois.guerard@univ-nantes.fr;
joelle.gaschet@univ-nantes.fr;
francois.davodeau@univ-nantes.fr

N. Chouin
INSERM UMR1232—CNRS UMR6299—Centre de Recherche en Cancérologie de Nantes-Angers (Equipe 13), Institut de Recherche en Santé de l'Université de Nantes, Nantes, France

AMaROC Research Group, ONIRIS (Nantes-Atlantic National College of Veterinary Medicine, Food Science and Engineering), Nantes, France
e-mail: nicolas.chouin@oniris-nantes.fr

M. Cherel
INSERM UMR1232—CNRS UMR6299—Centre de Recherche en Cancérologie de Nantes-Angers (Equipe 13), Institut de Recherche en Santé de l'Université de Nantes, Nantes, France

Department of Nuclear Medicine, ICO-René Gauducheau, Boulevard Jacques Monod, Saint-Herblain, France
e-mail: Michel.Cherel@univ-nantes.fr

M. Bourgeois
INSERM UMR1232—CNRS UMR6299—Centre de Recherche en Cancérologie de Nantes-Angers (Equipe 13), Institut de Recherche en Santé de l'Université de Nantes, Nantes, France

Department of Nuclear Medicine, University Hospital, CHU de Nantes, Nantes, France

GIP Arronax, Saint-Herblain, France
e-mail: mickael.bourgeois@univ-nantes.fr

© Springer Nature Switzerland AG 2019
L. Giovanella (ed.), *Nuclear Medicine Therapy*, https://doi.org/10.1007/978-3-030-17494-1_8

80%, Hodgkin lymphoma occurs in 10% of cases, and T/NK cell lymphoma accounts for approximately 6% of all lymphomas. Among the most frequent B-cell lymphomas, the clinical practice subdivides pathologies by morphological and phenotypic aspects of B-cell like Diffuse Large B-Cell Lymphoma (DLBCL), Burkitt lymphoma, Extranodal marginal zone lymphoma of mucosa-associated lymphoid tissue (MALT lymphoma), mantle cell lymphoma, or follicular lymphoma (FL).

Patient outcomes have improved greatly over the last 40 years as a result of the use of radiotherapy in cases of localized pathology, but mainly by multi-agent chemotherapy, immunotherapy, and stem cell transplantation. The guideline for treatment protocol choice is commonly based on the lymphoma subtype and the molecular signature for each of them. Over the last two decades, improvements in the information on the lymphoma phenotype have allowed targeted use of monoclonal antibodies (mAbs) in immunotherapy in combination with classical chemotherapy. While this has considerably improved the patients' prognosis and treatment, relapsed and refractory disease remain a major treatment challenge.

Lymphoma cells are well known to be radiosensitive and consequently are ideal targets for radioimmunotherapy (RIT) [2–4]. RIT is a targeted therapy, whereby irradiation from radionuclides is delivered to a tumor using monoclonal antibodies (MAbs) specifically directed to a tumor antigen, and can therefore be effective in patients who do not respond to nonradioactive "cold" immunotherapy.

8.2 General Principles of RIT

RIT is a cytotoxic approach which involves both immunological and radiobiological processes [5]. The RIT methodology relies on a radionuclide vectorization, or targeting, that is driven by the mAb specificity to a particular tumor antigen, with an irradiation of healthy tissues as low as reasonable. The internal irradiation generated by RIT presents the following benefits in comparison to conventional external beam radiotherapy: heterogeneous and continuous irradiation, and an exponentially decreasing low dose rate [6]. Currently, the mechanisms underlying this type of radiobiological irradiation are imperfectly known, and the dose-response relationship with patient outcomes, such as cell survival, has not yet been demonstrated. Despite these shortfalls, the synergy between the immunological cytotoxicity and RIT, including bystander and abscopal effects, is well established with a higher efficacy against the tumor [7].

The first clinical trial for chemotherapy-resistant non-Hodgkin's lymphoma was reported in 1988 by De Nardo et al., and used an anti-HLA-DR Lym-1 monoclonal antibody radiolabeled with iodine-131 [8]. RIT efficacy is mainly dependent on the mAb and isotope choice. Regarding therapeutic applications, nuclear medicine practitioners use massive emission particles such as beta-negative particles, Auger electrons, or alpha particles. These radioactive emission types specifically deliver their ionizing energy locally. The penetration distance of these radioactive emissions depends on the initial energy and should match the targeted tumor size. The path-length penetration for Auger electrons is of the order of a few nanometers and requires an internalization of the radiolabeled mAb to obtain efficient irradiation. For alpha particles, irradiation occurs up to several hundred micrometers around the emission point. For beta-negative particles, irradiation extends up to a few millimeters and results in a cross-fire effect on nearby tumor cells. This cross-fire effect may result in an antitumor effect against cells that are not specifically bound by the targeting mAb. Optimizing RIT requires a good balance between the pharmacokinetic/biodistribution properties of the mAb and the half-life of the radionuclides. To circumvent a potential mismatch, biochemists and immunochemists have developed a number of immunoconjugates which are derived from antibody molecules such as F(ab) and F(ab')$_2$ fragments or synthetic proteins (e.g., minibodies or single chain variable fragments) [7].

Today, the efficacy of RIT for the treatment of hematological cancers like lymphomas has been demonstrated and found to be beneficial for relapsed or refractory lymphomas or as consolidation after immunochemotherapy [9]. Despite evidence of clinical efficacy, RIT treatment remains limited in routine lymphoma therapy. The contrast between efficiency and current clinical use is probably due to the competition with other nonradioactive therapies and the necessity for RIT phase III randomized clinical trials to convince the oncohematologist community.

8.3   Efficacy of RIT in Lymphomas

As outlined above, the proof of concept study for RIT in non-Hodgkin's B-cell lymphoma used an anti-HLA-DR Lym-1 antibody radiolabeled with iodine-131 [8]. Because of the very large phenotypic variability in the lymphoma subtypes, RIT approaches have mainly focused on identifying and targeting the overexpressed antigen specific for each pathology subtype [10].

8.3.1   Anti-CD20 RIT

CD20 is an activated-glycosylated phosphoprotein expressed on normal B-cells, and is overexpressed in many B-cell lymphoma subtypes. Two radioimmunoconjugates targeting the CD20 antigen have been approved: ^{131}I-tositumomab (Bexxar®; GlaxoSmithkline) which was subsequently discontinued for commercial reasons and ^{90}Y-ibritumomab tiuxetan (Zevalin; Spectrum Pharmaceuticals) which continues to be used both in the USA and in Europe. The benefits of anti-CD20 ^{90}Y-ibritumomab tiuxetan in consolidation after induction in first-line therapy have been shown for follicular lymphoma, mantle cell lymphoma, and DLBCL patients [11–16].

Zevalin®, the only commercially available anti-CD20 RIT drug, is classically administered 6–8 days after a pre-dose of cold anti-CD20 mAb (2 × 250 mg of rituximab), which targets the same antigen as the RIT, in order to improve the biodistribution of the radioactive mAb. The posology of Zevalin® is based on patient body weight and platelet count. The therapeutic dose is classically 14.8 MBq/kg (0.4 mCi/kg) and 11.1 MBq/kg (0.3 mCi/kg) with a platelet count of 100,000–149,000/mm^3 [17].

Clinical results showed that Zevalin® and Bexxar® had a significant efficacy, but moderate response duration as monotherapy in rituximab-refractory recurrence of FL. RIT with anti-CD20 mAbs could be integrated into clinical practice using non-ablative doses for treatment of patients with relapsed or refractory FL, or as consolidation after induction chemotherapy. A meta-analysis of four clinical trials involving relapsing B-cell lymphoma patients treated by Zevalin® demonstrated a long-term response (time progression >12 months) in 37% of patients. The estimated 5 year overall survival (OS) was 53% for all patients treated with Zevalin® and 81% for long-term responders.

Recent studies have shown an increased efficacy where RIT was administered in combination with chemotherapy to obtain a myeloablative state. These approaches require autologous or allogeneic SCT. A recent prospective multicenter study consisting of Zevalin® administration (14.8 MBq/kg) in association with BEAM polychemotherapy (Carmustine/Etoposide/Cytarabine/Melphalan) demonstrated safety and efficacy in comparison with the BEAM protocol alone as a conditioning regimen for stem cell transplantation (SCT) in 43 patients with relapsed/refractory non-Hodgkin lymphoma. An international and randomized phase III clinical trial aiming to assess the benefits for RIT in first-line indolent advanced follicular lymphoma (FIT trial) [18] enrolled 414 patients with partial or complete response after standard front-line chemotherapy regimens. The 208 patients in the RIT arm (14.8 MBq/kg) of this large broad clinical trial showed a conversion rate of 77% from partial to complete response. After 3.5 years of follow-up, the median progression-free survival was significantly improved from 13.3 to 36.5 months. Patients in the RIT arm presented a greater than 5 year improvement in the time to next treatment. A long-term follow-up of these patients included in the FIT trial [19] confirmed these patient outcomes in terms of treatment consolidation with durable 19% progression-free survival advantage at 8 years and an improvement of the time to next treatment of 5.1 years for patients with advanced follicular lymphoma.

Hematological toxicity is the major side effect of RIT and depends on the extent of bone marrow involvement and prior treatment. Non-hematological toxicity is generally low. Secondary myelodysplastic syndrome (MDS) or acute myelogenous leukemia (AML) are rare symptoms and were reported in 1–3% of cases [11, 12, 15, 16]. In the FIT trial, MDS or AML was reported for seven patients in the RIT arm which enrolled 208 patients (3.4%) compared to one MDS in the control arm. Cytogenetic testing revealed chromosomal abnormalities typical of therapy-induced MDS/AML and confirmed the known risk increment in patients previously treated by several lines of chemotherapy or radiotherapy. Finally, the FIT trial didn't show additional long-term toxicities or congenital malformations [19].

8.3.2 Anti-CD22 RIT

CD22 is a transmembrane glycoprotein expressed on mature B-cells but not on stem cells or plasma cells. CD22 is expressed highly on a number of malignant B-cell lymphomas. It is also a relevant alternative target for B cell lymphomas which do not express the CD20 antigen or for patients with no response to cold anti-CD20 immunotherapy. The anti-CD22 mAb epratuzumab is a humanized mAb that has been extensively tested in RIT. It is internalized by the target cells and can be administered without the requirement for cold dose antibody pre-treatment such Zevalin® or Bexxar® [20].

^{90}Y-epratuzumab RIT has been developed as a repeat injection therapeutic. A multicenter study enrolled 64 patients with different B-cell lymphoma histologies. These patients were injected with activities ranging from 0.185 to 1.665 GBq/m^2 over several doses. The objective response rate was 62% (48% complete response/unconfirmed complete response). For FL subtype patients without SCT, response increased with total injected activity to 92% complete response/

unconfirmed complete response at higher dose (>1.11 GBq/m^2). Grade 3–4 hematological toxicities were observed and were manageable with support for patients with <25% bone marrow involvement.

An alternative to increasing the total administered dose without any additional hematological toxicity consists of a dose fractionation approach (see dose fractionation in RIT optimization part) [21, 22]. Using this approach, efficacy was demonstrated in a multicenter phase I/II study where patients with documented B-cell NHL received 92.5–1110 MBq/m^2 per injection repeated twice at 2–3 weeks intervals in a dose escalation protocol. For the highest doses the total dose administered was higher than in the classical single dose protocol. The adverse effects remained manageable (mainly grade 1–2 hematologic toxicity for low doses and frequently grade 3–4 for doses >740 MBq/m^2) and no abnormal pattern of changes occurred in standard serum chemistry. A fractionated approach for anti-CD22 RIT provides a high rate of durable complete response in relapsed/refractory NHL, and 740 MBq/m^2 injected twice at 2 week intervals seems to be a good efficacy/safety compromise [23]. More recently, the efficacy of RIT fractionation with CD22 targeting was confirmed for post-chemotherapy adjuvant treatment in diffuse large B-cell lymphoma (DLBCL) where patients were treated with two doses at 7 day intervals of 555 MBq/m^2 of ^{90}Y-epratuzumab tetraxetan (anti-CD22 mAb) [24].

This methodology demonstrated efficacy (no progression of the disease after standard chemotherapy) without acute toxicity (only grade 3–4 thrombocytopenia and neutropenia) [23].

8.3.3 Anti-CD37 RIT

CD37 is an internalizing transmembrane antigen overexpressed in most B-cell malignancies. The anti-CD37 mAb lilotomab has recently been used to treat indolent non-Hodgkin B-cell lymphoma (NHL) by RIT. For this application, lilotomab is pre-activated with a chelating agent (DOTA = satetraxetan) and radiolabeled with a bêta emitter such ^{177}Lu.

A phase I clinical trial with four arms [25] was designed to test pre-dosing regimens (one rituximab dose and two doses of cold lilotomab) to improve the safety and efficacy profile. In this study, patients with relapsed incurable NHL of follicular grade I–IIIA, marginal zone, mantle cell, lymphocytoplasmic, and small lymphocytic subtypes (all patient have platelet counts >150 × 10^9/L) were eligible for inclusion. A total of 36 patients were enrolled. The overall tumor response rate observed in 23 patients evaluable for efficacy was 57%, comprising 30% complete responses, 26% partial responses, 22% stable disease, and 22% with progressive disease. Furthermore, one patient is still in remission more than 3 years after treatment, and two patients are still in remission more than 2 years after treatment.

Hematological toxicity is the most common for all dose-limiting toxicities. Observed thrombocytopenia and neutropenia are reversible and manageable. A pre-dosing injection of nonradioactive lilotomab at a dose of 40 mg/m^2 reduces the incidence of hematological side effects for 15 MBq/kg of ^{177}Lu-lilotomab satetraxetan. A 100 mg/m^2 pre-dosing injection of non-radioactive lilotomab further reduces the red-marrow absorbed dose and to an increment of tumor/red-marrow ratio [26]. The dosimetry of ^{177}Lu-lilotomab satetraxetan for other critical organs (liver, spleen, and kidneys) was found to be modest in comparison to assumed tolerance limits [27, 28]

8.3.4 Anti-Tenascin RIT

Tenascin is a hexameric glycoprotein localized in the extracellular matrix. The tenascin-C variant is involved in tumor processes and in particular in the lymph nodes of B-cell NHL and HL [29, 30] but also in T-cell NHL [31].

A phase I/II clinical trial with 2.05 GBq/m^2 injection of ^{131}I-81C6 (anti-tenascin antibody) in eight refractory Hodgkin lymphoma patients was designed [29]. For refractory NHL, a phase I trial study enrolled nine patients with a dose regimen of 1.11 GBq or 1.48 GBq [30].

For Hodgkin lymphoma indication, at the first response assessment (4–6 weeks after therapy), one patient showed a complete response, one patient showed partial response, and five had disease stabilization. For non-Hodgkin lymphoma, one patient showed a complete remission and one a partial remission.

For Hodgkin lymphoma indication, only one patient developed grade IV thrombocytopenia and leukocytopenia. All other patients had hematological toxicity of grade III or lower. For non-Hodgkin lymphoma, one patient which received 1.48 GBq developed hematological toxicity that required stem cell infusion

8.3.5 Other Antigens Under Preclinical Development

The advances in lymphoma phenotypic discrimination and the knowledge and success of anti-CD20 immunotherapy have led to a large effort in identifying and exploring alternative molecular targets.

The CD74 antigen is the gamma chain of the MHC class II invariant chain, also known as Li fragment, and is expressed classically on the B-cell surface. CD74 is expressed at low levels but is rapidly internalized. This important turnover of CD74 molecules conduces to an important accumulation of anti-CD74 mAb in the B-cell lymphoma which will be used in RIT to accumulate intracellularly large amount of radioactivity. In this way anti-CD74 RIT with beta-negative or Auger electron emitters in Burkitt's lymphoma in vitro cultured cells showed specific and effective cytotoxicity [32].

The cell surface receptor CD30, also known as tumor necrosis factor receptor superfamily 8 (TNFRSF8), is physiologically expressed in activated T- and B-cells and is pathologically overexpressed in both T- and B-cell lymphomas. An anti-CD30 mAb, HeFi-1 conjugated to yttrium-90 appeared very promising in a B-cell lymphoma murine model, with tumor growth significantly inhibited compared to the control group [33]. More recently, CD30 was targeted using a ^{89}Zr radiolabeled antibody for phenotypic imaging and showed specific accumulation of the mAb in a murine xenograft model of T-cell non-Hodgkin's lymphoma [34, 35].

CD38 is a transmembrane glycoprotein over-expressed in multiple myeloma and other B-cell malignancies. Green and colleagues used a pre-targeting strategy (see Sect. 4.1 pretargeting approach) to study a murine model of NHL, and used a bispecific antibody directed against both CD38 and ^{90}Y-biotin [36]. This CD38 bispecific pretargeted RIT approach resulted in 75–80% complete remission at day 12 with minimal toxicity.

CD19 is a transmembrane glycoprotein anti-gen belonging to the immunoglobulin family and is expressed on all B-cells except for plasma and follicular dendritic cells. An in vivo study of a Burkitt's lymphoma xenograft murine model showed an antitumor activity for a single anti-CD19 mAb dose of 11.1 MBq, and most mice survived over 119 days with no evidence of tumors [37].

8.4 RIT Optimization

8.4.1 Pretargeting Approach

The key requirement for success of RIT relies on the ability to deliver the maximum radioisotope emission to the tumor while exposing healthy tissues to as little irradiation as possible. The pretar-geting approach consists of a two-step procedure. First, a bispecific cold (nonradioactive) mAb is administered; this mAb binds directly to the tumor target. The second injection delivers a low-molecular-weight radioactive hapten with a high affinity for the bispecific mAb which is bound to the tumor. The small size of the radioactive hap-ten allows both rapid tumor penetration and fast elimination of the unbound radioactivity from the body by renal clearance. The proof of concept for this strategy was first shown in a preclinical murine NHL model in 2018 [36].

8.4.2 Dose Fractionation

As described previously, the major limitation of RIT treatment for lymphomas is hematological toxicity. Dose fractionation in RIT is of interest because it allows healthy bone marrow regenera-tion to occur faster than tumor cell growth. This differential phenomenon in repair kinetics between healthy and cancerous tissues is well known in conventional external beam radiother-apy. For this purpose, a rationale for using frac-tionated doses with a total dose augmentation was reported in 2002 [38]. The first confirmation of this dose fractionation efficacy was reported using ^{90}Y-ibritumomab tiuxetan (Zevalin®) in 74 patients treated for FL (international phase II study—FIZZ study). The patients in this study received two doses of 11.1 MBq/kg at 8–12 week intervals for a 48% higher total dose compared to the classical single dose protocol [39, 40]. The results of this study demonstrated an improve-ment in overall response (94% vs. 87% for the single dose protocol) with a similar toxicity pro-file. Thus, the fractionation approach was clini-cally validated with a progression-free survival of 40 months versus 26 months for single dose treatment.

8.4.3 Other Isotopes

Despite the great number of radioisotopes that could be used in clinical RIT practice, only a few of them are currently used, the beta emitters iodine-131 and yttrium-90. The recent produc-tion and development of new isotopes raises the opportunity of delivering ionizing energy directly within tumors. Thus, for beta particle emitters, new isotopes such as lutetium-177 or copper-67 exhibit good irradiation parameters and promise improved benefits for patient outcomes [41–44]. On the other hand, alpha particle emitters such as astatine-211 or actinium-225 deliver a high pro-portion of their energy inside the targeted cells leading to highly efficient killing. Radiobiologic studies have demonstrated that 1–20 cell nuclei traversals by alpha particles are sufficient to inac-tivate a cell, compared to thousands or tens of thousands of beta-negative particles required to obtain the same effect. These physical radiobio-logic properties are particularly well suited for the purpose of treating hematological diseases such as lymphomas.

8.4.4 Diagnostic and Dosimetry Approach by Phenotypic Imaging

While mAbs play a pivotal role in RIT, they are also critical in the modern era of in vivo whole body phenotypic imaging. This complementary information can be acquired using Positron Emission Tomography (PET) technology where the mAb is radiolabeled with a beta-positive emitter [45]. A number of radioimmunoconjugates developed for PET imaging have been described, and these permit a precise phenotypic diagnosis and a dosimetric evaluation for RIT [46–48].

Radiation dosimetry studies using ^{89}Zr, a positron emitter, coupled to an anti-CD20 mAb such as rituximab [49] or the newly FDA approved obinutuzumab and ofatumumab [50] have demonstrated the efficacy of this application to localize the tumor site, estimate the therapeutic doses required in connection to dosimetric information, and follow the RIT efficacy in terms of tumor reduction.

8.5 Concluding Remarks

Relapsed and refractory NHL represents a significant challenge in medical care of lymphomas. In this indication, RIT has been successfully utilized with encouraging clinical results. RIT showed significant results in B-cell lymphoma, but moderate response duration as a monotherapy in rituximab-refractory B-cell lymphoma. The therapeutic impact may be higher when using RIT in a myeloablative approach, as consolidation after chemotherapy or as first-line treatment. The dose-limiting toxicity of RIT is hematological, and depends on bone marrow involvement and prior treatment.

Some progress in RIT, such as the fractionation approach, needs to be confirmed by comparative studies, but it seems to be appropriate for response consolidation after induction chemotherapy in older patients with advanced DLBCL. RIT appears to be relevant in the personalized medicine era where the targeted and multimodality strategy requires dedicated treatment for a poor-prognosis cancer that is resistant to conventional therapies. After a proof of concept phase in the 1990s and 2000s and many recent advances, it is now time for the oncohematology community as a whole, to assess the efficacy of RIT using randomized and stratified clinical trials and to adopt new protocols (new lymphoma antigens, fractionation, and pretargeting approaches), new isotopes (alpha- or beta-negative emitters), and improved pathology knowledge and phenotypic imaging.

Acknowledgments This work has been supported by the French National Agency for Research called Investissements d'Avenir via grants Labex IRON n ANR-11-LABX-0018-01 and Equipex Arronax plus n ANR-11-EQPX-0004.

References

1. Swerdlow SH, Campo E, Pileri SA, Harris NL, Stein H, Siebert R, et al. The 2016 revision of the World Health Organization classification of lymphoid neoplasms. Blood. 2016;127(20):2375–90.
2. DeNardo SJ, DeNardo GL, O'Grady LF, Macey DJ, Mills SL, Epstein AL, et al. Treatment of a patient with B cell lymphoma by I-131 LYM-1 monoclonal antibodies. Int J Biol Markers. 1987;2(1):49–53.
3. Press OW, Leonard JP, Coiffier B, Levy R, Timmerman J. Immunotherapy of non-Hodgkin's lymphomas. Hematology Am Soc Hematol Educ Program. 2001:221–40.
4. Cheson BD. Radioimmunotherapy of Non-Hodgkin lymphomas. Blood. 2003;101(2):391–8.
5. Pouget J-P, Lozza C, Deshayes E, Boudousq V, Navarro-Teulon I. Introduction to radiobiology of targeted radionuclide therapy. Front Med (Lausanne). 2015;2(4):12.
6. Pouget J-P, Navarro-Teulon I, Bardies M, Chouin N, Cartron G, Pèlegrin A, et al. Clinical radioimmunotherapy-the role of radiobiology. Nat Rev Clin Oncol. 2011;8(12):720–34.
7. Bourgeois M, Bailly C, Frindel M, Guerard F, Cherel M, Faivre-Chauvet A, et al. Radioimmunoconjugates for treating cancer: recent advances and current opportunities. Expert Opin Biol Ther. 2017;17(7):813–9.
8. DeNardo SJ, DeNardo GL, O'Grady LF, Hu E, Sytsma VM, Mills SL, et al. Treatment of B cell malignancies with131I Lym-1 monoclonal antibodies. Int J Cancer Suppl. 1988;41(S3):96–101.
9. Chao MP. Treatment challenges in the management of relapsed or refractory non-Hodgkin's lymphoma—novel and emerging therapies. Cancer Manag Res. 2013;5:251–69.

10. Merli M, Ferrario A, Maffioli M, Arcaini L, Passamonti F. Investigational therapies targeting lymphocyte antigens for the treatment of non-Hodgkin's lymphoma. Expert Opin Investig Drugs. 2015;24(7):897–912.

11. Bennett JM, Kaminski MS, Leonard JP, Vose JM, Zelenetz AD, Knox SJ, et al. Assessment of treatment-related myelodysplastic syndromes and acute myeloid leukemia in patients with non-Hodgkin lymphoma treated with tositumomab and iodine I131 tositumomab. Blood. 2005;105(12):4576–82.

12. Horning SJ, Younes A, Jain V, Kroll S, Lucas J, Podoloff D, et al. Efficacy and safety of tositumomab and iodine-131 tositumomab (Bexxar) in B-cell lymphoma, progressive after rituximab. J Clin Oncol. 2005;23(4):712–9.

13. Hohloch K, Lankeit HK, Zinzani PL, Scholz CW, Lorsbach M, Windemuth-Kieselbach C, et al. Radioimmunotherapy for first-line and relapse treatment of aggressive B-cell non-Hodgkin lymphoma: an analysis of 215 patients registered in the international RIT-Network. Eur J Nucl Med Mol Imaging. 2014;41(8):1585–92.

14. Hohloch K. Radioimmunotherapy of lymphoma: an underestimated therapy option. Lancet Haematol. 2017;4(1):e6–7.

15. Hohloch K, Delaloye AB, Windemuth-Kieselbach C, Gómez-Codina J, Linkesch W, Jurczak W, et al. Radioimmunotherapy confers long-term survival to lymphoma patients with acceptable toxicity: registry analysis by the International Radioimmunotherapy Network. J Nucl Med. 2011;52(9):1354–60.

16. Czuczman MS, Emmanouilides C, Darif M, Witzig TE, Gordon LI, Revell S, et al. Treatment-related myelodysplastic syndrome and acute myelogenous leukemia in patients treated with ibritumomab tiuxetan radioimmunotherapy. J Clin Oncol. 2007;25(27):4285–92.

17. Bodet-Milin C. Radioimmunotherapy of B-cell non-Hodgkin's lymphoma. Front Oncol. 2013;3:177.

18. Morschhauser F, Radford J, Van Hoof A, Vitolo U, Soubeyran P, Tilly H, et al. Phase III trial of consolidation therapy with yttrium-90-ibritumomab tiuxetan compared with no additional therapy after first remission in advanced follicular lymphoma. J Clin Oncol. 2008;26(32):5156–64.

19. Morschhauser F, Radford J, Van Hoof A, Botto B, Rohatiner AZS, Salles G, et al. 90Yttrium-ibritumomab tiuxetan consolidation of first remission in advanced-stage follicular non-Hodgkin lymphoma: updated results after a median follow-up of 7.3 years from the International, Randomized, Phase III First-LineIndolent trial. J Clin Oncol. 2013;31(16):1977–83.

20. Sharkey RM, Brenner A, Burton J, Hajjar G, Toder SP, Alavi A, et al. Radioimmunotherapy of non-Hodgkin's lymphoma with 90Y-DOTA humanized anti-CD22 IgG (90Y-Epratuzumab): do tumor targeting and dosimetry predict therapeutic response? J Nucl Med. 2003;44(12):2000–18.

21. Lindén O, Hindorf C, Cavallin-Ståhl E, Wegener WA, Goldenberg DM, Horne H, et al. Dose-fractionated radioimmunotherapy in non-Hodgkin's lymphoma using DOTA-conjugated, 90Y-radiolabeled, humanized anti-CD22 monoclonal antibody, epratuzumab. Clin Cancer Res. 2005;11(14):5215–22.

22. Bodet-Milin C, Kraeber-Bodéré F, Dupas B, Morschhauser F, Gastinne T, Le Gouill S, et al. Evaluation of response to fractionated radioimmunotherapy with 90Y-epratuzumab in non-Hodgkin's lymphoma by 18F-fluorodeoxyglucose positron emission tomography. Haematologica. 2008;93(3):390–7.

23. Morschhauser F, Kraeber-Bodéré F, Wegener WA, Harousseau J-L, Petillon M-O, Huglo D, et al. High rates of durable responses with anti-CD22 fractionated radioimmunotherapy: results of a multicenter, phase I/II study in non-Hodgkin's lymphoma. J Clin Oncol. 2010;28(23):3709–16.

24. Kraeber-Bodéré F, Pallardy A, Maisonneuve H, Campion L, Moreau A, Soubeyran I, et al. Consolidation anti-CD22 fractionated radioimmunotherapy with (90)Y-epratuzumab tetraxetan following R-CHOP in elderly patients with diffuse large B-cell lymphoma: a prospective, single group, phase 2 trial. Lancet Haematol. 2017;4(1):e35–45.

25. Kolstad A, Madsbu U, Beasley M, Bayne M, Illidge T, O'Rourke N, et al. Lymrit 37-01: updated results of a phase I/II study of 177Lu-Lilotomab satetraxetan, a novel CD37-targeted antibody- radionuclide-conjugate in relapsed NHL patients. Hematol Oncol. 2017;35:269–70.

26. Stokke C, Blakkisrud J, Løndalen A, Dahle J, Martinsen ACT, Holte H, et al. Pre-dosing with lilotomab prior to therapy with 177Lu-lilotomab satetraxetan significantly increases the ratio of tumor to red marrow absorbed dose in non-Hodgkin lymphoma patients. Eur J Nucl Med Mol Imaging. 2018;45(7):1233–41.

27. Blakkisrud J, Løndalen A, Dahle J, Turner S, Holte H, Kolstad A, et al. Red marrow-absorbed dose for non-Hodgkin lymphoma patients treated with 177Lu-Lilotomab satetraxetan, a novel anti-CD37 antibody-radionuclide conjugate. J Nucl Med. 2017;58(1):55–61.

28. Blakkisrud J, Løndalen A, Martinsen ACT, Dahle J, Holtedahl JE, Bach-Gansmo T, et al. Tumor-absorbed dose for non-Hodgkin lymphoma patients treated with the anti-CD37 antibody radionuclide conjugate 177Lu-Lilotomab Satetraxetan. J Nucl Med. 2017;58(1):48–54.

29. Aloj L, D'Ambrosio L, Aurilio M, Morisco A, Frigeri F, Caraco C, et al. Radioimmunotherapy with Tenarad, a 131I-labelled antibody fragment targeting the extradomain A1 of tenascin-C, in patients with refractory Hodgkin's lymphoma. Eur J Nucl Med Mol Imaging. 2014;41(5):867–77.

30. Rizzieri DA, Akabani G, Zalutsky MR, Coleman RE, Metzler SD, Bowsher JE, et al. Phase 1 trial study of

131I-labeled chimeric 81C6 monoclonal antibody for the treatment of patients with non-Hodgkin lymphoma. Blood. 2004;104(3):642–8.

31. Gritti G, Gianatti A, Petronzelli F, De Santis R, Pavoni C, Rossi RL, et al. Evaluation of tenascin-C by tenatumomab in T-cell non-Hodgkin lymphomas identifies a new target for radioimmunotherapy. Oncotarget. 2018;9(11):9766–75.

32. Govindan SV, Goldenberg DM, Elsamra SE, Griffiths GL, Ong GL, Brechbiel MW, et al. Radionuclides linked to a CD74 antibody as therapeutic agents for B-cell lymphoma: comparison of Auger electron emitters with beta-particle emitters. J Nucl Med. 2000;41(12):2089–97.

33. Zhang M, Yao Z, Patel H, Garmestani K, Zhang Z, Talanov VS, et al. Effective therapy of murine models of human leukemia and lymphoma with radiolabeled anti-CD30 antibody, HeFi-1. Proc Natl Acad Sci U S A. 2007;104(20):8444–8.

34. Moss A, Gudas J, Albertson T, Whiting N, Law C-L. Abstract 104: preclinical microPET/CT imaging of 89Zr-Df-SGN-35 in mice bearing xenografted CD30 expressing and non-expressing tumors. Cancer Res. 2014;74(19 Suppl):104.

35. Rylova SN, Del Pozzo L, Klingeberg C, Tönnesmann R, Illert AL, Meyer PT, et al. Immuno-PET imaging of CD30-positive lymphoma using 89Zr-desferrioxamine-labeled CD30-specific AC-10 antibody. J Nucl Med. 2016;57(1):96–102.

36. Green DJ, O'Steen S, Lin Y, Comstock ML, Kenoyer AL, Hamlin DK, et al. CD38-bispecific antibody pretargeted radioimmunotherapy for multiple myeloma and other B-cell malignancies. Blood. 2018;131(6):611–20.

37. Vallera DA, Elson M, Brechbiel MW, Dusenbery KE, Burns LJ, Jaszcz WB, et al. Radiotherapy of CD19 expressing Daudi tumors in nude mice with Yttrium-90-labeled anti-CD19 antibody. Cancer Biother Radiopharm. 2004;19(1):11–23.

38. DeNardo GL, Schlom J, Buchsbaum DJ, Meredith RF, O'Donoghue JA, Sgouros G, et al. Rationales, evidence, and design considerations for fractionated radioimmunotherapy. Cancer. 2002;94(4 Suppl):1332–48.

39. Illidge TM, Mayes S, Pettengell R, Bates AT, Bayne M, Radford JA, et al. Fractionated ⁹⁰Y-ibritumomab tiuxetan radioimmunotherapy as an initial therapy of follicular lymphoma: an international phase II study in patients requiring treatment according to GELF/BNLI criteria. J Clin Oncol. 2014;32(3):212–8.

40. Scholz CW, Pinto A, Linkesch W, Lindén O, Viardot A, Keller U, et al. (90)Yttrium-ibritumomab-tiuxetan as first-line treatment for follicular lymphoma: 30 months of follow-up data from an international multicenter phase II clinical trial. J Clin Oncol. 2013;31(3):308–13.

41. Kameswaran M, Pandey U, Dhakan C, Pathak K, Gota V, Vimalnath KV, et al. Synthesis and preclinical evaluation of (177)Lu-CHX-A″-DTPA-rituximab as a radioimmunotherapeutic agent for non-Hodgkin's lymphoma. Cancer Biother Radiopharm. 2015;30(6):240–6.

42. DeNardo GL. New directions in radioimmunotherapy of non-Hodgkin's lymphoma. Clin Lymphoma. 2004;5(Suppl 1):S4.

43. DeNardo GL, DeNardo SJ, Kukis DL, O'Donnell RT, Shen S, Goldstein DS, et al. Maximum tolerated dose of 67Cu-2IT-BAT-LYM-1 for fractionated radioimmunotherapy of non-Hodgkin's lymphoma: a pilot study. Anticancer Res. 1998;18(4B):2779–88.

44. DeNardo GL, Kennel SJ, Siegel JA, DeNardo SJ. Radiometals as payloads for radioimmunotherapy for lymphoma. Clin Lymphoma. 2004;5(Suppl 1):S5–10.

45. England CG, Rui L, Cai W. Lymphoma: current status of clinical and preclinical imaging with radiolabeled antibodies. Eur J Nucl Med Mol Imaging. 2016;44(3):517–32.

46. Knowles SM, Wu AM. Advances in immuno-positron emission tomography: antibodies for molecular imaging in oncology. J Clin Oncol. 2012;30(31):3884–92.

47. Boerman OC, Oyen WJG. Immuno-PET of cancer: a revival of antibody imaging. J Nucl Med. 2011;52(8):1171–2.

48. van Dongen GAMS, Visser GWM, Lub-de Hooge MN, de Vries EG, Perk LR. Immuno-PET: a navigator in monoclonal antibody development and applications. Oncologist. 2007;12(12):1379–89.

49. Natarajan A, Gambhir SS. Radiation dosimetry study of [(89)Zr]rituximab tracer for clinical translation of B cell NHL imaging using positron emission tomography. Mol Imaging Biol. 2015;17(4):539–47.

50. Yoon JT, Longtine MS, Marquez-Nostra BV, Wahl RL. Evaluation of next-generation anti-CD20 antibodies labeled with zirconium 89 in human lymphoma xenografts. J Nucl Med. 2018;59(8):1219–24.

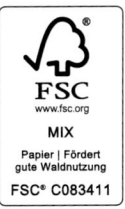